Care of the Dying Child

Edited by

ANN GOLDMAN

CLIC Consultant in
Paediatric Palliative Care

Great Ormond Street Hospital for
Children NHS Trust, London

WITHDRAWN

WITHDRAWN

Oxford   New York   Tokyo
OXFORD UNIVERSITY PRESS

Oxford University Press, Great Clarendon Street, Oxford OX2 6DP

Oxford   New York
Athens   Auckland   Bangkok   Bogota   Buenos Aires   Calcutta
Cape Town   Chennai   Dar es Salaam   Delhi   Florence   Hong Kong   Istanbul
Karachi   Kuala Lumpur   Madrid   Melbourne   Mexico City   Mumbai
Nairobi   Paris   São Paolo   Singapore   Taipei   Tokyo   Toronto   Warsaw

and associated companies in
Berlin   Ibadan

Oxford is a trade mark of Oxford University Press

Published in the United States
by Oxford University Press, Inc., New York

First published 1994
Reprinted (with corrections and updates) 1998

British Library Cataloguing in Publication Data
Data available

Library of Congress Cataloging in Publication Data

1 3 5 7 9 10 8 6 4 2

ISBN 0 19 261983 7

Typeset by Advance Typesetting Ltd, Oxfordshire

Printed in Great Britain on acid free paper by
Bookcraft (Bath) Ltd,
Midsomer Norton, Avon

Preface

Fortunately, death in childhood is uncommon, but for those families who have to confront the problems of caring for a terminally ill child, the burden is great. For the health care workers too, dealing with the particular problems of the dying child and their family, as well as acknowledging and coming to terms with their own sadness, can provoke considerable stress and anxiety.

It has taken many years for society, including the medical profession, to acknowledge the problems of dying patients. Although the adult hospice movement is well established, it is still relatively young. In paediatrics, where death is less common, it is only now becoming clear that terminally ill children and their families have special needs which are often not recognized or met. In part, this is a reflection of the relatively small numbers involved, but it is also a result of the discomfort most of us feel when facing the certain death of children. Compared with other aspects of paediatrics, there is very little written about terminal care in children. Although we can learn from the growing literature of the adult hospice movement, the problems are not identical; children need to be considered in their own right and appropriate skills and expertise developed to help them.

The intention of this book is to identify the medical, psychological, and practical issues of caring for terminally ill children and their families, and provide a source of current knowledge in the field. It focuses on children with chronic disease, and the specific issues of perinatal death, sudden infant death, accidental death, and suicide are not addressed. The aim of the book is to be of help to paediatricians and family doctors in particular, but also to other professionals who may be involved in caring for a dying child. I hope it will help them to look after the children with skill and confidence, and work with and support the families so the children can die in peace and with dignity, whether at home or in hospital.

Acknowledgements

My thanks go to all the authors for their written contributions but also to some for their moral support, others for their patience, and others for their struggle. I hope they will feel it was justified. I am grateful too, for the time and interest of many other colleagues; I have benefited from their experience and knowledge. In particular, my thanks to Ann Ayres, Sharon Beardsmore, Angela Bowman, June Dyer, Maggie Fitzpatrick, Mary Goodwin, Anne Hunt, Sarah Lederman, Susan Madge, and Jeanette Singer. My special thanks also to Jean Mancini for her skill, tolerance, and willing help with all the typing. For my financial support and their interest in the work I am pleased to acknowledge the Welton Foundation.

Contents

Contributors

Derek Bacon, BA, M.Sc, DAC, CACP
Faculty of Social Health, Sciences and Education, University of
Ulster, Coleraine, Londonderry BT52 1SA
Formerly Hospital Chaplain, Great Ormond Street Hospital for
Children, Great Ormond Street, London WC1N 3JH

David Baum, MA, MSC, MD, FRCP
Professor of Child Health, Institute of Child Health, Royal Hospital
for Sick Children, St Michael's Hill, Bristol BS2 8BJ

Dora Black, MB, FRC.Psych.
Honorary Consultant Child and Adolescent Psychiatrist,
Traumatic Stress Clinic, 73 Charlotte Street, London W1P 1LB

Roger Burne, MB, BS, MRCCP, D.Obst. RCOG
St Bartholomew's Medical Centre, Cowley Road, Oxford OX4 1XB

Candy Duggan, RGN, RSCN, RHV
Clinical Nurse Specialist for HIV/AIDS, South Park Clinic,
South Park Drive, Ilford IG3 9AN

Ann Goldman, MA, MB, FRCP
CLIC Consultant in Paediatric Palliative Care, Great Ormond Street
Hospital for Children, Great Ormond Street, London WC1N 3JH

Richard Lansdown, Ph.D, FBPsS, C.Psychol
Honorary Senior Lecturer in Psychology, Institute of Child Health,
Guilford Street, London WC1N 3EH

Philip Rees, B.Sc, FRCP, DCH
Consultant Paediatric Cardiologist, Great Ormond Street Hospital
for Children, Great Ormond Street, London WC1N 3JH

Jean Simons B.A. (Hons), MSC, CQSW
Bereavement Services Co-ordinator, Great Ormond Street Hospital
for Children, Great Ormond Street, London WC1N 3JH

Alan Stein, MB, BCh. MRC.Psych
Leopold Muller Professor of Child and Family Mental Health,
Leopold Muller University Department, Royal Free Hospital,
Pond Street, London NW3 2QG

Avril Trapp, D.Ed, CQSW
Formerly: Senior Sargent Social Worker, Royal Victoria Infirmary,
Queen Victoria Road, Newcastle-upon-Tyne NE1 4LP

Helen Woolley BA, PSW
Research Associate, Section of Child and Adolescent Psychiatry,
University of Oxford, Park Hospital for Children, Headington,
Oxford OX3 7TQ

1

Introduction:
the magnitude of the problem

David Baum

For most families living in western industrial societies, the concept of child mortality has been relegated to history. The improved living conditions in our cities, the effective delivery of clean water and removal of sewage, food in relative abundance, coupled with advances in medicine and science, all but promise each family a healthy outcome to conception, pregnancy, the birth, and development of their children. Nevertheless, although at levels unimaginably low even one generation ago, deaths in infancy and childhood do still occur.

The western world is uncomfortable with death, particularly death in childhood. In the United Kingdom today, the expectations of good health and the perceived curative powers of technological medicine, may actually serve to heighten the anguish of the families who lose their children. As fewer families experience mortality in childhood, there is a smaller pool of parents and professionals with the experience to support those whose children die or are afflicted with a mortal illness.

The parents feel cheated or deceived, and should the child die in hospital away from the family home, the grief is exacerbated by feelings of powerlessness and isolation from the emotional support network of the neighbourhood. A community with shared experience and wisdom is no longer available to sustain them through each day and through each crisis of bereavement in its turn.

No better prepared for death, but possibly more fatalistic in accepting it, families in earlier times were accustomed to infant mortality. Thus, Dr Johnson's friend, Mrs Thrale, gave birth to 12 children, only four of whom survived (Hyde 1977). While this is reported with sadness, it does not appear remarkable that the family is not overwhelmed by grief. Such conditions continue to prevail in industrially under-developed countries even today: in Ethiopia, for instance, half the children born each year will not live beyond their fifth birthday.

THE MAGNITUDE OF THE PROBLEM

The causes and nature of childhood death have changed over the years. In the United Kingdom and in most industrialized countries, accidents are currently the leading cause of death in childhood if one excludes death in the perinatal period and infancy. Cancers and leukaemias are in second place, followed by the more slowly progressive, rarer disorders such as muscular dystrophy, cystic fibrosis, mucopoly-saccharidoses, and miscellaneous neurodegenerative conditions (Table 1.1).

Broadly speaking, the deaths can be divided into those which occur suddenly, more or less unexpectedly (as with accidents, deaths in the perinatal period, sudden infant death syndrome, and overwhelming infections), and those deaths which the parents can anticipate, following either a life-limiting illness (one which is likely to progress and terminate life before adulthood as, for example, muscular dystrophy, cystic fibrosis, or mucopolysaccharidoses), or a

Table 1.1 Causes of death in childhood in broad categories, age 1–14 years in England and Wales in 1990 (HMSO 1990)

Accidents and poisoning	659
Malignancies	364
Infections	112
Others	934

life-threatening disease (one in which medical intervention may prove successful but by its nature carries a substantial chance of mortality in childhood as, for example, cancer and leukaemia, or conditions leading to major organ failure—heart, liver, kidney).

The recent report from ACT (Association for the care of Children with life threatening and terminal conditions and their families) and the RCPCH (Royal College of Paediatrics and Child Health) has suggested four groups of children who may need palliative care (Table 1.2).

Table 1.2 Children who may need palliative care

---

* Conditions for which curative treatment is possible but may fail.
* Diseases where premature death is likely but intensive treatments may prolong good quality life.
* Progressive conditions where treatment is exclusively palliative and may extend for many years.
* Conditions, often with neurological impairment, causing weakness and susceptibility to complications.

It has been difficult to quantify the mortality and morbidity figures accurately for children dying from life-threatening and life-limiting illnesses, particularly as these children have not been thought of as a cohesive group until recently. The most up-to-date information including data from voluntary societies, suggest the figure for the annual mortality rate for children aged between 1 and 17 years with life limiting conditions is 1 per 10 000 whilst the morbidity rate is approximately 10 per 10 000.

A useful way to look at this is to extrapolate the figures for a district of 250 000 people with a child population of approximately 50 000. In one year 5 are likely to die from a life-limiting condition, of which 2 would be from cancer, 1 from heart disease and 2 from other life limiting conditions. About 50 children would be suffering from a life-limiting condition at any one time and about half of these would be needing palliative care (While 1996).

The magnitude of the problem can be expressed in a number of ways; consider three possible models. Firstly, an estimate can be made of the prevalence of individual conditions across the nation. This is shown in the maps (Figs 1–5) together with population density figures to illustrate the relative rarity of the conditions and potential isolation of the families at a district and regional level.

The second model is derived from the patterns of usage of the existing children's hospices. The use of these beds for respite and terminal care by the affected families leaves no doubt as to the families' perception of their needs, and thereby offers some indication of the national burden in supporting families with children suffering progressive incurable diseases. Tables 1.3 and 1.4 refer to the use of beds in Helen House.

A third model looks at the progression of the family burden associated with life-threatening and life-limiting conditions (Fig. 1.6). While there is insufficient information available to truly calculate the currency of the need in this way, it is clear, in drawing the area under such a curve, that the needs of the family and the child in the early phase of the condition are different from the needs emerging in the middle phase, and again from those of the post-terminal phase. One could imagine constructing similar curves to reflect the cumulative needs of such families at a regional or national level by extrapolation from national prevalence figures and the usage of the existing caring facilities.

THE DIVERSITY OF NEEDS

For each child and his or her family, the ordeal begins with the identification of a life-limiting or life-threatening disorder; family values and plans must undergo radical changes and a phase of bereavement is initiated. At this stage, the family needs expert medical care and counselling by those familiar with the particular condition. A particular difficulty that many such families encounter is the relative rarity of the disorder which may be outside the knowledge and experience of their primary care team and indeed of the locally based specialists. This opens up a dimension to family needs which in some cases persists till the death of the

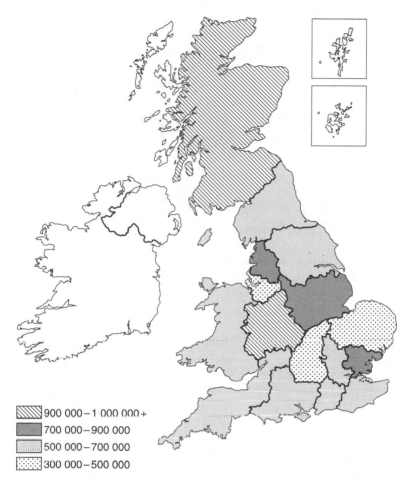

Fig. 1.1 Population of children in England, Scotland, and Wales, aged 0–14 in 1988 (HMSO, 1990). Total child population = 10 364 962.

child, namely, that appropriate experience in treatment and symptom relief is available at a distant specialist centre or through the collective experience of a parent-led self-help group or society, rather than through their own doctor or hospital.

These children may suffer from slowly or rapidly progressive disorders. Their clinical management and underlying

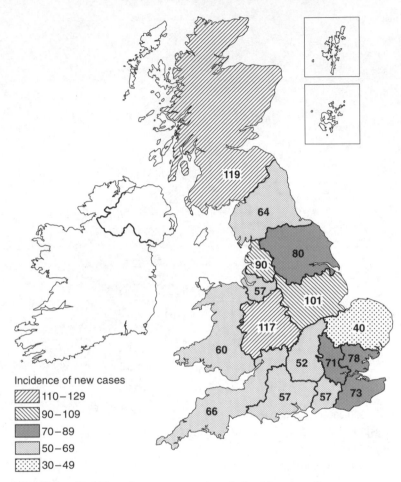

Fig. 1.2 Childhood cancer: annual incidence of new cases (UKCCSG). Total = 1181 (1 in 10 000 children).

pathological problems are hugely diverse. Their symptomatology varies between groups and individuals, and within individuals across the passage of time and progression of their disease. As the disorder progresses, the needs of the child and family will be affected by the speed of change and the particular manifestations of the disease, whether it be loss of muscular power, as with the muscular dystrophies,

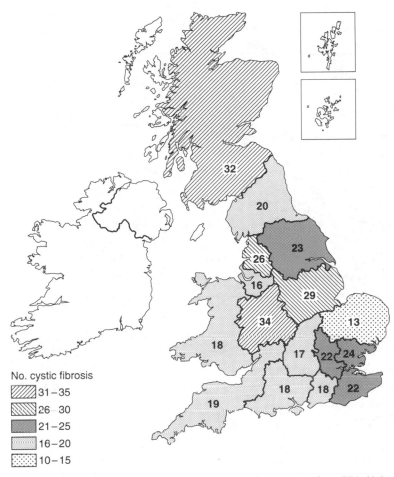

Fig. 1.3 Cystic fibrosis: annual birth incidence. Total = 351 (1 in
2000 births).

neurodegenerative problems and dementia, as with the
mucopolysaccharidoses, vital organ failure with intermittent
crises associated with organ transplantation, or the infiltra-
tive effects of a leukaemia or cancer resulting in bone marrow
suppression or pain, coupled with the noxious side-effects of
chemotherapy and radiation treatment. During this varied
and highly individual phase of disease progression, children

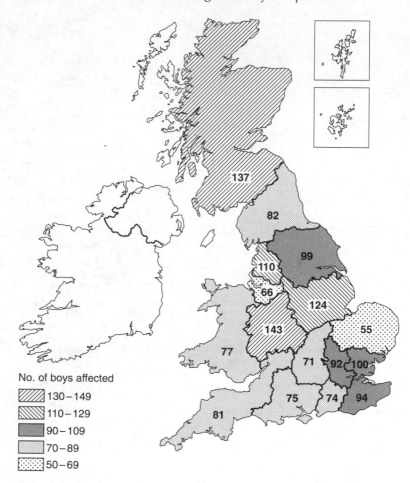

No. of boys affected

- 130–149
- 110–129
- 90–109
- 70–89
- 50–69

Fig. 1.4 Duchenne's muscular dystrophy: prevalence. Total = 1470 (1 in 3500 boys).

and their families suffer physical, emotional, spiritual, and financial stresses, and potential exhaustion.

The care of the terminal phase of illness in such children, the management of their anticipated death, and the care of the family, neighbours, and friends after the child's death are matters of accruing experience. Generally speaking, the view expressed by those whose children have been referred to children's hospices (approximately one-third of whom die

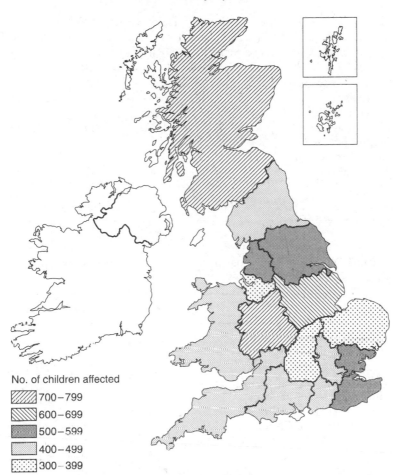

No. of children affected

- ⚏ 700–799
- ⚏ 600–699
- ⚏ 500–599
- ⚏ 400–499
- ⚏ 300–399

Fig. 1.5 Prevalence of children with rare, miscellaneous life-threatening disorders (Contact-A-Family, 1989). Total = 8000.

within 12 months of referral) is that the child should die at home if possible and if appropriate care is available. Individually, however, family circumstances and particular symptom problems may render this inappropriate or impossible.

The diverse, particular and uncommon needs of these children and their families have led to the development of a national association, ACT (Association for the care of

Table 1.3   Reasons for admission to Helen House, 1988–90

	1988	1989	1990	Mean
Planned respite	258	228	257	248
Holiday	30	53	40	41
Social occasion	5	12	1	6
Unplanned respite	7	5	14	9
Family illness	11	8	8	9
Symptom control	8	6	10	8
Terminal care	1	4	2	2
Other	27	17	16	20
Total	347	333	348	343

Table 1.4   New admissions each year to Helen House by diagnostic categories, 1988–90

	1988	1989	1990
Cerebral tumours	1		
Other tumours		4	1
Neuromuscular	5	1	4
CNS degenerative	16	4	3
Mucopolysaccharidoses	8		
Congenital abnormalities	1	4	2
Non-progressive CNS disease	3	6	2
Cystic fibrosis	1		
Metabolic	5	1	1
Others		1	1
Total	40	21	14

children with life-threatening or terminal conditions, and their families) to serve as a resource to advise on available services, to serve as advocate for the needs of each child and family, and to influence government planning in favour of a comprehensive service, including hospice and respite care, for children throughout the country. As an instrument of service to individual families, the national association has developed a charter.

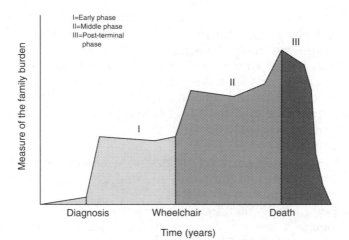

Fig. 1.6   A model expressing the needs of a hypothetical child with muscular dystrophy and his family progressing over the years.

ACT CHARTER FOR CHILDREN WITH LIFE-THREATENING OR TERMINAL CONDITIONS AND THEIR FAMILIES

1. Every child shall be treated with dignity and respect, and shall be afforded privacy whatever the child's physical or intellectual ability.
2. Parents shall be acknowledged as the primary carers, and shall be centrally involved as partners in all care and decisions involving their child.
3. Every child shall be given the opportunity to participate in decisions affecting his or her care, according to age and understanding.
4. Every family shall be given the opportunity of a consultation with a paediatric specialist who has particular knowledge of the child's condition.
5. Information shall be provided for the parents, and for the child and the siblings, according to age and understanding. The needs of other relatives shall also be addressed.

6. An honest and open approach shall be the basis of all communication which shall be sensitive and appropriate to age and understanding.
7. The family home shall remain the centre of caring whenever possible. All other care shall be provided by paediatric trained staff in a child-centred environment.
8. Every child shall have access to education. Efforts shall be made to enable the child to engage in other childhood activities.
9. Every family shall be entitled to a named key worker who will enable the family to build up and maintain an appropriate support system.
10. Every family shall have access to flexible respite care in their own home and in a home-from-home setting for the whole family, with appropriate paediatric nursing and medical support.
11. Every family shall have access to paediatric nursing support in the home, when required.
12. Every family shall have access to expert, sensitive advice in procuring practical aids and financial support.
13. Every family shall have access to domestic help at times of stress at home.
14. Bereavement support shall be offered to the whole family and be available for as long as required.

SUMMARY

Meeting the needs of families with mortally afflicted children is not a statistical or definitional issue; each family needs care and support appropriate to its particular circumstances. The fact that the child's condition is common or rare is significant only in so far as it affects the availability of appropriate expertise and the organization of appropriate caring and support services.

The care and support required by children with life-threatening illnesses and their families varies according to the child's particular disease and its progression, and according to each family's coping abilities and their individual psychological and financial resources. The child's needs range from treatment and symptom relief, to education, recreation, affection, and access to a pattern of living similar to his or her friends, with all its challenges and rewards. Family and professionals alike need to see the youngster as a child first, and a patient second.

We have only begun to recognize the magnitude and diversity of the problems that face children with mortal illnesses and their families. While we may hope to see the therapeutic fruits of laboratory research improve the prognosis and reduce the morbidity from such conditions in the years to come, for the immediate future it remains our responsibility to give a proper place to palliative care paediatrics and to secure the appropriate provision of family support services nationwide to meet the needs of every family as set out in the ACT Charter.

REFERENCES

Association for children with life-threatening or terminal conditions and their families (ACT) and Royal College of Paediatrics and Child Health (RCPCH) (1997). *A guide to the development of Children's Palliative Care Services.*

Hyde, M. (1977). *The Thrales of Streatham Park.* Harvard University Press.

HMSO (1990). *1990 Mortality Statistics OPCS,* Series DH6 No. 4. London.

While, A., Citrone, C., Cornish, J. (1996). *Executive Summary. A study of the needs and provisions for families caring for children with life limiting incurable disorders.* Department of Health Publication.

2

Different illnesses and the problems they cause

Ann Goldman

Acknowledging that every child and family are unique and will approach their child's illness and death in their own way is important. Nevertheless, some of the child's symptoms and the problems and feelings the family will experience are shared by others in similar situations. Later chapters develop these common psychosocial issues, specific symptoms and their management in more detail. This chapter looks separately at some of the illnesses which cause death most frequently in children, and what particular pattern of problems can be anticipated for these children and their families. HIV and AIDS is considered in more detail because of its newness and potential importance in the future.

MALIGNANT DISEASE

The outlook for children with malignant disease continues to improve, and two-thirds can expect to be cured. However, at the time of diagnosis, each family has to face the knowledge that their previously well child now has a life-threatening disease. Many parents' knowledge of cancer is scant and may be inappropriately assumed from experience with elderly relatives. Fears of treatment, side-effects, and the inevitability of death are common.

The majority of children with malignant disease are cared for at specialist centres. The needs of families for support, from the time of diagnosis, through treatment and particularly at times of relapse and terminal illness, have been well recognized.

Multidisciplinary teams have been established at the centres including play specialists, psychologists, and social workers as well as medical and nursing staff, to provide both the children and their families with help in these areas.

Particular care needs to be taken to establish good communication links when a child's care is shared between a regional centre, local hospital, and primary health-care team. In recent years the development of home-care teams and liaison nurses has helped towards this. They also play an important role for families when a child is terminally ill, enabling them to be cared for at home by providing support and experience in symptom management.

Most of the children dying from malignant disease die from progression and spread of their tumour, but a small percentage die from complications of treatment aimed at curing the disease. The terminal care of these two groups of patients is different. Those for whom cure is still a possibility, are likely to be in hospital and receiving intensive supportive treatment, whereas for those with progressive disease with no likelihood of cure, the emphasis of treatment will have changed, and be palliative. Families have time together, and some possibility of making plans and choices.

Stopping treatment

When a child with malignant disease relapses, the oncologist and family are faced with the decision of whether to continue with treatment directed against the tumour or focus on palliative care. Many factors may influence this choice, including the chance of achieving further remissions, the oncologist's personal approach, and the family's own feelings. For some families, if no cure is possible then giving the child a short period of life without unpleasant therapy is their preferred option, whereas others find it would be impossible to live with themselves in the future unless they had tried every last option.

Even when further treatment is instituted for a period, there almost always comes a time when the medical staff and family acknowledge that the child is not going to be cured of his cancer. Although discussing stopping treatment against the tumour and acknowledging that death is inevitable can be very difficult, it offers an opportunity to confront the situation openly. The stress of uncertainty is removed and problems can be anticipated and planned for.

Support

Time and support from a trusted and experienced professional, often the nurse from the home-care team, to talk through the situation is vital. Many factual questions need answers: what symptoms will he get? will she have pain? what can we give for it? can he die at home? who will help us? Other questions may not have answers but need exploring: how long will it be? can we cope? what shall we say to her? what about his brothers and sisters? Some questions are difficult to admit to, but most families experience them: how can we think about the funeral whilst she's still alive? is it wrong to wish it were all over? Also, the many and complex feelings which accompany these questions need considering and voicing. Whilst some families want information immediately and talk easily, others find it more difficult and build up a picture gradually as the child's condition changes. The staff need to be as flexible as possible and respond to each family individually.

Symptoms

The symptoms which a child dying from cancer develops will depend on the sites of disease, both primary and metastatic. The type of symptoms that children with cancer develop terminally are similar to those in adults but, because of the different range of tumours children suffer, some of these assume a greater importance.

Pain is a significant problem for the majority of children. In a recent study, 87 per cent of children dying from progressive malignant disease required opioid analgesics. Although a number of these children (17 per cent) needed them for less than 24 h, 70 per cent required them for longer. Direct involvement of tissue by tumour deposits is the most common cause of pain, and this may be of bone, bone marrow, or soft tissues. Distension of organ capsules or obstruction of tissues may also give rise to pain. These pains tend to be dull and aching in nature but can be severe. Sometimes the nature of the pain suggests invasion or compression of a nerve and is stabbing or burning in nature. It is possible to provide good relief of pain for the majority of children although there are some for whom it is not complete. Neurogenic pain in particular can be resistant.

Gastrointestinal symptoms including nausea, vomiting, constipation, and sore mouth, are frequently seen. Careful assessment to elicit the cause is important so that the most appropriate treatment can be instituted. Although anorexia often occurs in terminally ill children, the severe cachexia seen in adults is not common, which may be a reflection of the shorter length of children's terminal illnesses. Children with large mediastinal tumours or lung secondaries, particularly from osteogenic sarcoma, may have problems from dyspnoea. Fortunately, this is a less common problem than in terminally ill adults.

Many childhood tumours, particularly leukaemias and neuroblastoma involve the bone marrow in the terminal stages. Potential problems from this include anaemia, thrombocytopenia, and infections as well as widespread bone pain. It is possible to provide both platelet and red cell transfusions over many months and there can be a dilemma about whether to do so.

Red cell transfusions can offer a child improved quality of life when his or her symptoms are primarily being caused by anaemia. Careful discussion with the family is important so that they appreciate that although transfusions may be appropriate at one point in a child's care, there is likely to come a point as the disease progresses when the quality of life has declined and transfusions are no longer helpful or felt to be appropriate.

During chemotherapy, it may have been routine to transfuse according to platelet level, but in palliative care, platelets can be reserved for bleeding problems which interfere with the quality of life, such as persistent nose bleeds or haematemesis, but not petechiae. However, for children with a strong history of bleeding problems during their illness such as those with acute promyelocytic leukaemia, regular platelet transfusions may be planned.

Brain tumours make up one-fifth of all childhood primary tumours. The course of the terminal disease for these children is often more prolonged. Potential symptoms include vomiting and headaches caused by raised intracranial pressure. Convulsions may also occur. Progressive neurological deterioration with motor defects, and feeding and communication problems can be distressing.

Conclusion

Families of children with cancer need the opportunity to choose where to care for their child. They need to know that wherever that may be, home, hospital, or hospice, they will have skilled, sympathetic help to manage the child's symptoms, to support them all, and that working together to ensure the child's comfort and dignity will be the aim of all the staff involved.

PROGRESSIVE DEGENERATIVE DISEASES
Roger Burne

As the prognosis for children suffering from malignant diseases improves, the relative importance of progressive degenerative diseases as a cause of death in childhood increases. With few exceptions, the outlook for children with these conditions has not improved. These conditions which have been gathered together here, present a clinically diverse group with an enormous range of neurological, neuromuscular, metabolic, and other clinical features. Table 2.1 reflects the range, showing the diagnoses of the children seen at Helen House between 1982 and 1989. Cystic fibrosis and Duchenne's muscular dystrophy are relatively well known with a higher incidence, and are discussed separately. Individually, the diagnoses are rare although collectively they account for a considerable number of children. The unifying features are the progressive and inexorable deterioration, the inevitability of early death, and, in most cases, an inherited cause.

Table 2.1 Specific diagnoses of 154 children admitted to Helen House, suffering from progressive degenerative conditions, in the period 1982–89

CNS degenerations	
Undiagnosed CNS degenerations	20
Batten's disease	19
Adrenoleucodystrophy	6
Metachromatic leucodystrophy	5
Sub-acute sclerosing panencephalitis	4
Leigh's encephalopathy	3
Other	12
	69
Mucopolysaccharidoses	
Sanfillipo syndrome	27
Hurler's syndrome	6
Hunter's syndrome	5
Other	1
	39
Neuromuscular	
Duchenne's muscular dystrophy	21
Spinal muscular atrophy	7
Other	2
	30
Metabolic	
Cystic fibrosis	3
Other	9
	12
Epidermolysis bullosa	3
Fibrosing alveolitis	1

'Other' includes diagnoses where there were only one or two children.

The time of diagnosis

In most of the degenerative conditions, only general sup-portive care is possible from the time of diagnosis. This bleak prospect is one which the child's parents will have had to live with from the time that the diagnosis was made. In a very real sense, both the terminal phase and indeed bereave-ment start at the time that the inevitability of death is conveyed. This gives particular importance to the way in which the diagnosis of such major conditions is communi-cated to parents. Even many years later, the time of diagno-sis remains a vivid memory for most parents. A significant number remain dissatisfied with the way the information was given to them. Parents appreciate being given the diagnosis as soon as possible in an open and sympathetic way; they wish to be seen in private and be uninterrupted, with the opportunity to ask questions and receive replies in clear, understandable language. Most parents welcome early information about the disease, its causes, and its pro-gression.

After such news has been conveyed, clear arrangements must be made both for the care of the child and to allow further discussion and questions. The provision of informa-tion about appropriate self-help groups can be a great help at this time. They can provide contact, advice, and help over the months and years of illness which are to follow. This group of families, with the prospect of many years of caring for their children, need and value respite care and the support of children's hospices.

This initial phase is given emphasis here because it is likely to be a powerful influence on the events which are to follow. Parents who are given the diagnosis in a helpful way, who are offered information about the disease, who receive appropriate follow-up and services, and who are advised of the possibilities for self-help, will be in a much better situation to cope with the end stages of the illness, than will parents who have been less well treated.

Inherited conditions

Particular problems may arise in relation to those conditions which are inherited. The commonest method of inheritance is autosomal recessive (e.g. cystic fibrosis and most mucopolysaccharidoses). The other common method of inheritance encountered is X-linked recessive (e.g. Duchenne's muscular dystrophy, Hunter's syndrome). In both cases, the initial diagnosis needs to be followed by urgent provision of genetic counselling. The timing of diagnosis assumes particular importance in those conditions which may not present for months or even years after birth. Any delay in establishing an accurate diagnosis may result in the delivery of a brother or sister with a risk of sharing the inherited condition. With speed, accuracy of diagnosis, and the increasing scope and accuracy of antenatal diagnosis, this risk can be minimized but not, unfortunately, eliminated. Twins who both have the same condition will continue to be born, as will babies whose elder siblings have not yet manifested their condition. This means that there continue to be families who have more than one child with the same progressive condition.

The fact that a child has inherited a fatal condition as a result of abnormal genes from one or both parents provides a fertile ground for feelings of guilt and self-blame. This factor needs to be kept in mind when communicating the diagnosis and throughout the course of the illness.

Symptom management

All these conditions are rare and, except in the most highly specialized centres, doctors in general practice or even a consultant paediatrician may have little or no direct personal experience. Frequently, with time, the parents possess a great depth of technical knowledge. This can result in a situation when doctors or nurses may be reluctant to venture an opinion on treatment, even when it is appropriate for them to do so. It must be remembered that children with unusual conditions present with 'normal' illnesses just as often as their healthy siblings and require just the same treatment. When complications of the underlying degeneration occur, then advice can readily be obtained from specialist centres or from appropriate charities or self-help groups.

Frequently, the assessment of the severity of symptoms in these children is especially difficult. Not only do considerations of age and understanding apply, but many children suffer from brain damage or reduced intellect as a result of their condition. This puts the emphasis on careful and detailed observation of the child, and demands special attention to the opinions of the parents who may be the only people capable of interpreting the presence or severity of distressing symptoms.

Pain

Pain occurs for some children with progressive neuro-degenerative illnesses. It can be difficult to recognize and assess and should be evaluated and relieved as quickly as possible. Causes of pain include muscle spasm, reflux oesophagitis, constipation, and joint pains, which require treatments appropriate to the cause. It is not often severe, and opioids are seldom required though they should be used if necessary.

Epilepsy

Many of the degenerative conditions affect the central nervous system. This means that epilepsy is especially common and may have been a presenting symptom. Control of seizures in such children does not differ from that used in more conventional circumstances, with the use of one, or at the most two, anticonvulsants used at full dosage rather than smaller doses of a larger number of drugs. Increasing the number of anticonvulsants can just risk additional side-effects and interactions without improving control. The paradoxical situation can even arise where seizures diminish if the medication is gradually reduced. Progressive neuro-logical conditions can present difficulties because the nature, frequency, and severity of the fits can vary during the course of the condition. Changes in anticonvulsant medication may be needed to reflect this. Severe, long, and frequent fitting can sometimes occur.

Skin care

The care of pressure areas is not usually a problem in childhood, but the combination of prolonged immobility, gross deformity, and severe illness which may be encountered in chronic progressive disease increases the risk considerably. This problem is especially likely to occur in children with neurological conditions. The best management is to prevent their occurrence by scrupulous nursing care. Regular turning, possibly up to hourly, combined with care of the pressure areas is required. The child will usually be nursed on a sheepskin, while a Spenco, ripple mattress, or water-bed may be helpful.

Food and drink

Feeding problems are especially common in children with progressive degenerative conditions when they affect the neurological and neuromuscular mechanisms which are vital for swallowing. Any reversible local cause should be treated.

Sometimes, the feeding difficulties are simply a result of generalized weakness, and consideration should always be given to the possibility of a cause which would respond to acceptable treatment. In many children with fatal illnesses, the causes of feeding problems will not be amenable to treatment. Help for their problems must then be centred on symptomatic relief.

Children who are suffering from feeding problems cause considerable anxiety for their families and to carers. This requires patient explanation, discussion, and training. Realistic eating goals can be set for pleasure and comfort; nutritional goals aimed at the restoration or maintenance of health, are likely to be inappropriate. Perhaps most important is that time should be allowed for unhurried gentle and enjoyable feeding.

In general, frequent, small meals will be preferred. Careful attention to temperature, consistency and flavour are important. Hard or dry foods should be avoided and sometimes a purée is easier to swallow than a liquid. Solids should be cut into small bite-size pieces and may be moistened with gravy or sauce. Uncooked dairy foods tend to thicken mucus, and may be best avoided.

The child's position and surroundings must be carefully arranged to be correct for their individual needs and preferences. The head should be stabilized with the chin slightly tilted downwards. Gentle help to close the child's lips while chewing may be needed. The swallowing reflex can be helped by stroking the child's neck. The feeder should check that the last mouthful has been swallowed before giving another and should avoid scooping food off the child's chin with a spoon. There are a wide range of cups, spoons, plates, and other aids or appliances which may be of assistance. Choice of the right aid may prolong a child's ability to feed independently, or ease the difficulties of feeding the totally-dependent.

Tube feeding is often regarded as a distressing and invasive procedure. Although this may be true, it can be well tolerated by many children, provided that modern tubes are used. While a nasogastric tube will enable fluids, food, and drugs to be given, it will do nothing to alleviate the problems which may be caused by excess secretions and may make them worse. With improved surgical techniques, a gastrostomy can easily be fashioned and should be considered with the family if tube feeding is likely to be necessary for a prolonged time.

Any decision to assist feeding a child clearly needs very careful consideration and discussion with the family before they can come to a decision. Usually, it will be reserved for those cases where significant distress will be alleviated or where it will extend a child's useful or enjoyable life. It can be helpful to discuss these issues earlier rather than later, so that a considered policy may evolve gradually over a period of time.

MUSCLE DISORDERS

The variety of different muscle disorders which affect children can cause problems ranging from mild disability to those which are life-threatening. For some diseases, such as severe spinal muscular atrophy (SMA), death can be expected during infancy, whereas others, like Duchenne's muscular dystrophy develop and progress through childhood, with death as an adolescent anticipated. The majority of diseases are genetically determined and may be caused by progressive degeneration in the muscle cells themselves, specific structural or metabolic damage to the muscle cells, or as a secondary process resulting from degeneration of spinal anterior horn cells.

Since none of these diseases can be cured, care for the children is palliative from the time of diagnosis. Problems of mobility may dominate in the earlier stages but as the child gets older, or the disease progresses, feeding and breathing difficulties increase. The practical needs, problems of symptom management, and psychosocial issues are closely linked, and change and increase as the diseases progress. Families build up a large network of people involved in the care of their children, and co-ordination by a local key worker can be valuable. The Family Care Officers and the National Occupation Therapy Adviser, funded by the Muscular Dystrophy Group, provide a valuable resource for children with muscle disorders. Although their case-loads and the areas they cover are large, many are able to make home visits. They have expert knowledge and experience of the problems involved for families, and are able to offer valuable advice to them and to the professionals involved. They can also recommend any specific financial and practical help which may be available.

Problems in infancy

Children with major problems at an early age are characterized by those with spinal muscular atrophy (SMA,

Werdnig–Hoffmann). Parents are faced with the emotional distress and problems of the diagnosis of an incurable genetic disease from birth, and also have immediate and progressive physical problems to cope with. The majority of children die by the age of two years, but even giving as uncertain a prognosis as this, can be difficult for families, who may ask 'what did we do wrong?' if their child dies before the hoped-for two years.

Babies with SMA are not intellectually impaired. They have the curiosity of a normal baby but the inability, because of their severe weakness, to satisfy it. They have little strength to move their arms against gravity, and less in their legs, so they cannot explore or even put things into their mouths. This can make them quite demanding to care for.

Physically, they may be able to swallow and suck initially, but usually require assisted feeding later. Secretions become an increasing problem. Families benefit from having a small portable sucker (which can be acquired through the local authority) at home from an early stage. Hyoscine patches are a helpful and non-invasive way of reducing secretions. Recurrent chest infections occur and most children die from pneumonia. Many families prefer to nurse their child out of hospital as much as possible, and keep standby supplies of antibiotics at home. Others develop close ties to the local ward and come in and out at short notice as they need to.

Problems for older children

Duchenne's is the most common form of muscular dystrophy, with about 100 boys born annually and 1500 boys living with the disorder in the United Kingdom at any time. It is a genetically-determined (sex-linked recessive) progressive degenerative disorder, resulting from a defect in the protein dystrophin in muscle. There may be an associated cardio-myopathy and sometimes intellectual impairment.

The physical course of the disease is relentlessly downhill from the outset of symptoms within the first five years of life. Early management focuses on maintaining mobility with exercise, physiotherapy, and efforts to prevent contractures and spinal deformity. If these develop, treatment, including surgery, may be needed. The ability to walk is usually lost between the ages of eight and eleven. It may be prolonged for a short time with the use of leg calipers but eventually an electric wheelchair will be needed. Later, as the shoulder girdle muscles weaken, arm rests can be fitted to the wheelchair, to allow the boy to retain as much use of his hands as possible.

Eventually, even sitting and lying become uncomfortable. Even adjusting the bedclothes for themselves becomes impossible and disturbed nights for the boys and parents are routine. Electric beds with hand-controlled switches may help. Feeding themselves, chewing, and swallowing become increasingly difficult and weight loss is common over the last months.

Problems with chest infections become more frequent and more serious. They are the final cause of death for over two-thirds of the boys. Most families have antibiotics available at home and try to keep the children out of hospital if possible. However, recurrent admissions for treatment of pneumonia are usual. Most clinicians in the United Kingdom feel that the use of ventilators is not appropriate, but practice in other countries varies. Hypoventilation, especially at night, can cause headaches, nausea, and drowsiness during the day and restlessness at night. Oxygen through nasal prongs, either just at night or with top-ups during the day may relieve these symptoms. Cardiac disease accounts for a number of deaths. Occasionally these are sudden but often cardiac myopathy and damage to the lungs through recurrent infections result in increasing cardiac failure.

As normal a life as possible, for as long as possible is important for the emotional well-being of these boys. Encouraging them to develop interests within their capabilities can help reduce boredom and depression. Most attend local schools initially, but eventually they may need to go away to schools especially equipped to deal with their physical needs.

It is particularly difficult that their increasing handicap and dependence coincides with the teenage years when normally they would be becoming more independent. Maintaining dignity and privacy are virtually impossible. Ignorance and misunderstandings about the norms of physical and sexual development are common, as the boys are unable to explore their own bodies, and are not exposed to the physical contact or conversation of a normal peer group. These concerns can be frightening and embarrassing, and are often unspoken.

Both the parents and boys often become focused on physical aspects of care and become trapped in a system of mutual protection regarding the discussion of their emotions. At special schools where the children are faced with the deaths of friends, opportunities can be made for them to talk about their illness and feelings more openly; black humour abounds but mutual support is also possible.

CYSTIC FIBROSIS

When cystic fibrosis (CF) was first described in 1930, children died within the first few years of life. Although there is still no cure for the underlying abnormality, the prognosis has improved dramatically. Now three-quarters of those suffering from CF are still alive in their late teens and there are increasing numbers of adults.

The clinical features of the disease stem from abnormality of the exocrine system, with effects on the respiratory and digestive systems dominating and progressing with time. Comprehensive and lifelong care is essential to maintain a good quality life as long as possible. Supervision of care by specialist centres with multidisciplinary teams has been shown to improve life expectancy, and this is usually combined with shared care by a local paediatrician and the primary health care team. However, the responsibility and commitment for the time-consuming, unremitting, practical day-to-day care falls on the parents. The knowledge of the inevitability of premature death is with these families from the time of diagnosis, but in recent years, the end-point has become confused by the new possibility of heart–lung transplantation for some patients.

Physical problems

Regular physiotherapy, postural drainage, and exercise, combined with a variety of antibiotic treatments are employed to delay persistent lower respiratory tract infection and lung damage. Routine pancreatic enzyme replacement and good dietary intake, sometimes with additional aggressive supplementation, helps maintain good nutritional status. Unfortunately, inevitably as the disease progresses, problems develop; lung damage occurs, infections become increasingly difficult to treat and eventually cor pulmonale ensues. Symptoms linked with progressing disease include dyspnoea and cough, headaches, exhaustion, insomnia, and back and chest pain.

Pneumothoraces may occur as a feature of advanced lung disease, and although small ones may reabsorb spontaneously, intercostal drainage may be required for others, and if this fails, thoracic surgery may be needed. Haemoptysis is another frequent complication of advanced disease. Fortunately, it is usually only streaking and small clots of blood, but very occasionally, a massive bleed may occur as a terminal event.

Significant liver disease with problems of portal hypertension, hypersplenism, oesophageal varices, and jaundice occur in over 10 per cent of adolescents and adults. Haematemesis may then occur and the treatment of varices with sclerotherapy is made more complicated by the risks of anaesthesia, as these children are likely to have severe lung disease by this time.

Heart–lung transplants

The first heart lung transplant (HLT) was performed in 1985. It is only offered to those with very severe lung disease and a short life expectancy; about 50–60 patients each year might require assessment, and a number will not be considered appropriate. Physical contraindications include previous major thoracic surgery, invasive *Aspergillus* infection, severe malnutrition, and liver disease. It is also essential that a patient has a positive psychological approach and a history of good compliance with past treatments. Even after assessment and selection for the transplant list, a transplant is not guaranteed as insufficient donor organs are available. Many patients die 'on the list'.

Those children who have a successful HLT may experience a dramatic improvement; those who have been completely dependent on oxygen may return to work on education. However, there is a significant mortality to the procedure, continuing immunosuppressive treatment to counteract rejection is needed, and both the short- and long-term side-effects are still being discovered and assessed. Although patients may look to transplant as a cure it is still another, albeit dramatic, aspect of palliation.

As death approaches

At the moment, the majority of children with cystic fibrosis die in hospital. Most have developed a very close relationship with the ward and staff over many years and have great confidence and close friendships with them. A number of specialist nurses in cystic fibrosis now exist, who are able to go out into the community and advise and support families who decide that they would like terminal care at home, if possible.

In the past, as cystic fibrosis progressed, eventually the imminence of death was obvious and could be acknowledged, and care could focus on symptom relief. If the child is not eligible for transplantation this is still the case. However, after a lifetime of intensive treatment, it can be difficult to abandon past patterns of care. Often families prefer to gradually wind down, for example by continuing gentle physiotherapy whilst stopping antibiotics. Opioids can be given to relieve the distress of dyspnoea and coughing.

HLT has changed this for many families, and for staff too. In spite of the limitations of HLT, its possibility has meant that the need to acknowledge that death is inevitable can be postponed. The possibility of making plans about death, and for the family to grieve together, is lost as the active fight against the illness continues. Those children on the transplant list come straight back to hospital if their condition deteriorates, in the hope that intensive treatment might resolve the immediate crisis so that they can continue to wait for their transplant.

Psychological problems

These form a very significant part in the morbidity of the illness. Time must be spent in the early period after diagnosis helping the parents understand the physical details of the illness and the treatment. The shock and inevitable feelings that accompany the knowledge that their child has an inherited, lifelong and life-threatening illness must also be explored. The chronic, progressive, and debilitating nature of the illness make for many practical difficulties. Frequent visits to hospital for review, and admission for intensive treatments have implications in the time spent travelling, separations involved and absences from education and work. Depression in parents and marital breakdown are not uncommon. Parents will describe the exhaustion and apathy that can develop when they are 'grieving on an elastic band'. Others will talk of the strain as other children they know with cystic fibrosis die and they become 'professional funeral goers'.

The children themselves have to face increasing physical limitations and the frustrations these bring. They see their friends and fellow patients become increasingly ill and eventually die, and as they become older have an increasing insight into their own long-term prognosis. How they react to this may depend on their own personality and the family's coping patterns. Some may be increasingly anxious and fearful, others show tremendous strength and determination. They may be able to establish a pattern of openness with their friends and set a positive example, like the teenager who was dying and was able to say to her friend in the next bed 'You'd better have my boots now'.

The teenagers themselves often establish an unspoken pecking order, in which they anticipate who is likely to die next. An unanticipated death, out of order, can be particularly difficult to bear for the others. The awful sense of being next in line can also be imagined. Other particularly bad times for these families and children may be anticipated when the child is coming up to the age when a brother or sister died. Birthdays can also be a time of dread, when you can anticipate one year less of your life.

There is a particular tension for those awaiting transplant, hoping desperately that the bleep will go off. Even though the child is becoming more and more ill, the knowledge that the transplant may be round the corner makes it very difficult for patients and the staff to let go. It is only very rarely that a family are able to give back their bleeper, however ill the child becomes. If a transplant does occur, the euphoria that the staff feel for the patient is balanced by the depression from those families who didn't get the prize this time. Some new and interesting effects are becoming apparent for families where the child does receive a transplant. The time-consuming programmes of treatment that had become part of the pattern of family life need to change. The children are not used to the 'well' role and have never had to compete on normal terms. New expectations and relationships need to evolve within the family now that some of the allowances made for being a sick child within the family are withdrawn, although the possibility of graft rejection and complications of immunosuppressant drugs still hovers, threateningly.

LIVER DISEASE

Children can be affected by a range of serious liver diseases. Many are inherited disorders with no curative treatment available, although surgery, diet, and drugs may help control the situation. Unfortunately, many types of chronic liver disease are progressive and eventually fatal causing about 75 deaths in children each year, with the majority in children aged 4 years and under. Since the mid-1980s, transplantation has become possible and this has dramatically altered the pattern of care for children with irreversible liver damage, as well as the expectations of their families.

Today, there is rarely a clear end-point when the family know that death is inevitable and treatment moves clearly from intent to cure, to palliation. Throughout the course of the disease, much of the treatment is palliative in nature but, although the family are aware that the disease is life-threatening, there is also the awareness of the possibility of transplant in the distance.

Symptoms

The symptoms and signs of liver disease reflect the importance and range of functions of the liver. Among these are its role in digestion and carbohydrate metabolism, the production of bile, production of blood-clotting factors, its role in metabolism and detoxifying substances, and its importance in the immune processes. A failing liver can also result in damage to other organs particularly the brain and kidneys.

Jaundice

Jaundice may occur, and it is particularly severe if there is hypoplasia of biliary ducts. The child and family are often distressed by the child's appearance and feel stigmatized. Itching associated with cholestasis can be severe.

Bleeding

Serious bleeding is associated with the presence of portal hypertension and oesophageal varices. It is also exacerbated by low levels of clotting factors which increase the prothrombin time, and low platelets from hypersplenism. Haematemesis can be unpredictable and life-threatening. Until recently, major surgery was often undertaken but was frequently unsuccessful, but now treatment is by sclerosis of abnormal vessels with injection of ethanolamine via an endoscope. This may need to be undertaken regularly and over many years, and can result in oesophageal narrowing and reflux.

Neurological problems

Chronic neurological problems with learning difficulties, clumsiness, and progressive loss of skills occur in some children. This can be a particularly distressing symptom for families and also for older children with insight into their situation. The cause is not well understood but may be linked to damage from protein metabolites, so a low protein diet and lactulose may be recommended.

Acute encephalopathy can occur, with confusion, agitation, fits, and coma. This life-threatening problem can develop more gradually or be precipitated, for example by a sudden gastrointestinal bleed. Benzodiazepine drugs such as diazepam and midazolam can be helpful but chlorpromazine and haloperidol, which are hepatotoxic, should be avoided. Elective ventilation and paralysis may be needed in the acute situation.

Others

Ascites and oedema are common as liver disease progresses. Fluid restriction, spironolactone, and albumin infusions may help. Paracentesis is only a very temporary measure. Hypoglycaemia, if it is a problem, can usually be controlled through giving the child small and regular feeds either orally or nasogastrically. Anorexia, nausea, anaemia, fatigue, and growth failure can all be part of the picture for these children.

Transplants

In the past, severe progressive disease inevitably led to death, but now almost all families can be offered a transplant for their child. Uncontrolled ascites, uncontrolled bleeding, rising prothrombin time, decreasing quality of life, and serious lack of growth may all be indications for a transplant. Contra-indications are rare but include other organ damage, chronic Epstein–Barr (EB) virus, tumour outside the liver, and severe handicap. As the disease progresses, all families are included in the choice about whether to have a transplant. There is now about a 75 per cent survival but the surgery is major, lifelong immunosuppressive drugs are required afterwards, and long-term effects are still unknown. Almost all families opt for a transplant, since death is inevitable without, but nevertheless the decision can be agonizing. Families may find themselves crying not only for their own child but for the child who they know must have died when a liver becomes available.

The pattern of disease and the availability of transplants means that virtually all deaths from liver disease occur in hospital, whilst everyone is still striving to deal with a situation which they hope and believe can be altered. This may be awaiting transplant, during a crisis after surgery, during overwhelming fungal infection, or because of rejection of a transplant. Sometimes when it does become clear that death is certain, there may only be a very short time available for the family and staff to adjust. However, even in this situation it is possible to help the family by keeping them fully informed, including them in the child's care and offering them privacy and time together.

CARDIAC DISEASE
Philip Rees

Life-threatening cardiac problems are most often the result of congenital abnormalities which affect the structure of the heart, major blood vessels, or the vessels in the lungs. They may also develop later through primary cardiac muscle disease (cardiomyopathy) as a consequence of inflammation of coronary arteries (Kawasaki disease), after infectious diseases, or as a result of previous chemotherapy. They may also occur in association with other diseases such as cystic fibrosis or muscular dystrophy.

The overall aim for the child is to provide maximum quality of life, both physical and emotional, usually through active treatment. If possible, a complete surgical repair will be undertaken, if not, temporary improvement will be sought through palliative surgery and management of symptoms. In the past, if complete correction of the problem was not possible, the expectation would be of gradually increasing symptoms and eventual death. However, cardiac transplant is now possible and this has changed. Both families and staff now anticipate that as the disease progresses, or when it is very severe from the outset, cardiac transplant will be available.

This approach to treatment means that the majority of children who die from cardiac disease do so in an acute peri-operative or intensive care setting, related to surgical repair or transplants. A small group of children with chronic heart disease die suddenly and unexpectedly, probably related to arrhythmias. There are only a few situations in which everyone recognizes further aggressive treatment is no longer appropriate and the focus moves openly to terminal care.

Symptoms of chronic cardiac disease

These symptoms result from the inability of the heart to meet the needs of the body, by receiving and pumping out adequate supplies of blood. The symptoms may start gradually, usually related to increased body demands such as exercise, emotion, or intercurrent illness, but then progress to occur with minimal exercise or change in temperature, and eventually at rest. A number of different symptoms are common and a child may suffer from several at the same time.

Fatigue, weariness, and exhaustion are very frequent complaints and are associated with a poor blood supply to the skeletal muscles. Increasing breathlessness is also common as the heart is unable to supply sufficient oxygenated blood, and the resulting oxygen debt leads to an increased respiratory rate. Excess fluid accumulating in the lungs may exacerbate this problem.

Fluid often also collects in the abdomen, legs, and face as the heart is unable to cope with the volume of returning blood and the resulting high pressure leads to the leak of fluids through the vessel walls. Abdominal discomfort, nausea, and vomiting result from the enlarged liver, pressure on the stomach, and the poor blood supply to the bowel. Eventually this can result in reduced bowel motility and absorption of food with progressive weight loss.

Dizziness and fainting may occur as the heart is unable to meet the demands for cerebral blood supply, as well as through sudden changes in heart rhythm. Arrhythmias may also result in palpitations. Pain is not common, although occasionally cramp-like chest pain from ischaemia may occur, particularly with cardiomyopathies.

Management of symptoms

A number of general approaches aimed at reducing the demands on the heart may help. This might include limiting activity and helping mobility by providing a big buggy or electric wheelchair. Small volumes of interesting and varied food given frequently are more acceptable, and reducing excess fat which slows stomach emptying may help the nausea. Ensuring adequate rest is important and comfort may be improved with extra pillows. Some sedation such as temazepam at night may also help.

Drugs to relieve symptoms, even though the underlying cause cannot be altered, may improve the child's comfort; gentle diuretics which reduce fluid accumulation are helpful, although this must be balanced by the heart's need for a good filling pressure in order to work effectively; anti-emetics for nausea and vomiting, morphine for breathlessness and agitation, and diazepam for anxiety may also be useful. Oxygen may improve symptoms of dyspnoea, and headaches and drowsiness from hypoxia. It may be supplied through nasal prongs using a portable oxygen cylinder or overnight using an oxygen concentrator. These can be prescribed by the family doctor, but unfortunately are very expensive (over £2000 at present).

The majority of children are under the care of a cardiologist and they may introduce more specific drug therapies. Vasodilators such as captopril can reduce the blood pressure and cardiac muscle work; nifedipine can also help through vasodilation, increasing the blood flow through the lungs. The role of digoxin, to increase the force of contraction of the heart muscle, is debatable in this situation, but is coming back into fashion.

Heart transplants

Cardiac transplants can be offered for the majority of children so long as they have good lung arteries, good family support, and no other major physical or emotional problems. The results of heart transplant are improving, with 70 per cent of the children alive one and four years later. If problems occur, they tend to be acute and early. Those children who have had a heart transplant have a good quality of life, although they will all require immunosuppressive drugs long-term. Unfortunately, despite these drugs the new heart is likely to suffer low grade rejection. This is a major long-term worry as current treatments are unsatisfactory. As there is flexibility in the size of hearts which can be used for heart transplants, the donor pool is wider than for heart–lung transplants; 80 per cent of eligible patients get a suitable heart with an average waiting list of three months.

Heart and lung transplants are more recent. The waiting list is twelve months with only 60 per cent of the patients eventually being transplanted. The results from heart lung transplants are also not as good, and although 70 per cent of the children transplanted are alive at one year, by three years this has fallen to 60 per cent and continues to fall. Problems occur with chronic rejection and obliterative bronchiolitis, which reduce the child's quality of life, and those whose primary problem was cystic fibrosis will continue to have the other manifestations of the disease.

Psychosocial issues

For many people, the heart has a very special significance, symbolizing life and the centre of all emotions. This can make the anger, fear, and guilt feelings very powerful for the family at the time of diagnosis. If the baby is a good size and looks relatively well, it can be hard for parents to believe the seriousness of the diagnosis. Often everything happens very quickly with transfer to the special care baby unit, then to a cardiac centre, and then to theatre within days of birth. There may be a relatively short time to talk through the underlying illness, the implications of surgery, and the possibility of death.

For older children with more chronic disease, problems of isolation, anger, and depression may develop both for the families and the sick child. The principle of communication with the family is to maintain an honest and sensitive approach that allows the continuing trust of the child and also includes them as much as possible in the planning and management of their problem. Parents, children, and staff often cope by retaining a positive and fighting spirit which is helpful during the illness. Unfortunately, through doing this, they sometimes lose sight of the fact that the disease is potentially life-threatening and this can make communicating and acknowledging the approach of death difficult.

When death is inevitable

For a few children, both the staff and the family decide that aggressive treatment is not appropriate and everyone is aware that the child is terminally ill. This may happen in the situation of a neonate with inoperable disease, perhaps with multiple other problems, also for older children who are not suitable for a heart transplant, or a group of children who have had a heart transplant but developed complications afterwards. In this situation it may be possible to work with the family and the child, offering choice about where they would like to be cared for and having time to consider and face the emotional problems of the impending death.

For most children with cardiac disease, this is not a possibility, with aggressive intervention occurring right to the point of death, with the agreement of both the family and medical staff. However, even in these circumstances staff on the ward can help the family by offering privacy and time with the child's body afterwards, opportunities to talk through the situation and resolve any unanswered questions, and support and follow-up through their bereavement.

RENAL DISEASE

Although children continue to develop renal disease, since the introduction of dialysis and transplant programmes, deaths from end-stage renal failure are rare. Problems from renal disease have two peaks in children. The first group is infants born with severe congenital or genetic disease who

develop problems early. A second peak occurs in late childhood or early teens when renal function in those with
acquired disease has declined gradually and becomes critical.

In the past, all these children would have become pro-
gressively more ill and died from renal failure, but now
dialysis and transplantation is the routine treatment and
offered to virtually every child. Today, the majority of deaths
occur in hospital to children involved in an active treatment
programme and are a result of complications. Palliative care
is chosen only for a small number of children including those
who never embark on dialysis and transplantation, and
those who, having been through many years of intensive
treatment, eventually opt to discontinue it.

Choosing palliative care

The small group of children where a positive decision is
made not to begin dialysis and aggressive treatment, tends
to be those for whom renal disease is only one of many
problems. Children with congenital heart disease, multiple
other congenital abnormalities, and intellectual impairment
may be either physically or psychologically unsuited to the
intense and chronic nature of a dialysis and transplantation
programme. For these children, the specialized nephrology
centre in discussion with the family may choose palliative
care. The children and families usually then continue their
care jointly between the specialist centre, their local hospital,
and the primary health care team.

Dialysis and transplantation offer life-saving treatment for
renal failure. Results can be excellent, offering good quality
of life for many children, and encouraging both families and
professional staff. However, they do not provide a cure.
Many children continue to die in the acute hospital setting
from complications of treatment. Dialysis and transplantation is technically still difficult in children below 10 kg, and
the three-year graft survival for children less than five years
old is only 55 per cent compared with a 75 per cent five-year
graft survival for older children. Those children who receive
transplants and continue on immunosuppressive drugs,

are at increased risk of infections. If the transplant fails, they may need to go back on dialysis and await a further transplant. Some children have now had up to four transplants.

As children get older, many become dispirited by the chronic and debilitating nature of their illness and treatment. Normal school life and peer relations may be difficult. Many are very small and unhappy about their body image. Some adolescents become non-compliant and may occasionally refuse to continue on treatment, fully aware that this means they will die.

Symptomatic problems

It is very difficult to predict how long a child will live after such a decision has been made. Death may be very rapid and sudden, possibly from cardiac arrhythmia due to electrolyte imbalance, or the children may decline very gradually over many months and even years. In the child who has already been receiving treatment for chronic renal failure, dietary manipulation, correction of acidosis and salt-wasting, prevention of renal osteodystrophy, regular injections of erythropoietin and antihypertensive agents might all have been part of treatment as well as dialysis and transplantation. Consideration must be made of how tolerable these are for the child, which it might be appropriate to discontinue, and which it is appropriate and important to continue, to provide symptom relief.

As the disease progresses, nausea and vomiting are common, and result from uraemia. A high carbohydrate diet will reduce the uraemia and symptoms resulting from it, and this may need to be given via a nasogastric tube. Anti-emetics may also help. Pain is unusual but anaemia, with tiredness and weakness is common. Platelet dysfunction may occur and result in bleeding into the skin and gut. As renal function declines, further fluid overload with oedema and dyspnoea may be a problem and, associated with this, pericardial effusion and tamponade may be a terminal event. Other children may develop convulsions and eventually coma before death.

Support for the family

The decision to choose palliative care may be a very difficult one for families, particularly those whose child has been ill over many years when the family and medical team may have adopted a positive and pragmatic approach to the illness, putting aside consideration and discussion of its likely outcome as long as possible. It can be difficult both for the families and carers to balance optimism and encouragement with reality. The family are likely to need considerable support through the prolonged and very uncertain period of decline, especially as the links which they have had with the referral centre are likely to be reduced and links with local staff will need to be built up.

FURTHER READING

Brett, E. (1991). *Paediatric neurology*. Churchill Livingstone, Edinburgh.

Dinwiddie, R. (1990). Cystic fibrosis. In *The diagnosis and management of paediatric respiratory disease*, pp. 177–222. Churchill Livingstone, Edinburgh.

Dubowitz, V. (1995). *Muscle disorders in childhood*. Saunders, London.

Mowat, A. (1994). *Liver disorders in childhood*. Butterworth-Heinemann, Oxford.

Plowman, N. and Pinkerton, R. (ed.) (1997). *Paediatric oncology–clinical practice and controversies*. Chapman & Hall, London.

HIV AND AIDS
Candy Duggan

Since 1994 there have been major developments in diagnosis and the treatment for children with HIV infection. However, no cure has been found and HIV is still surrounded by a powerful aura of fear and stigma, both for families and for some professionals. Working with families with HIV and AIDS confronts each of us with profound issues of living and dying. We have to examine our deepest fears, our beliefs, and our values. It presents some special issues, different from other chronic life-threatening illnesses. Some of these are because of its nature; it is an unpredictable illness with a wide spectrum of clinical problems, some of which are very uncommon. Differences also occur because HIV/AIDS is a family disease (Gibb *et al.* 1991) with more than one family member affected. Even paediatric staff used to working with the chronically ill have rarely had to deal with the possibility of concurrent illness and death of the child and his or her mother, father, and siblings.

EPIDEMIOLOGY

AIDS was first reported in children in 1982 in the USA, and in 1984 in Europe. It has been estimated that there are over one million children affected with HIV, world-wide (Chin 1990). Many of the earliest cases resulted from the use of infected blood in transfusions, and in blood products given to haemophiliacs. Since screening and heat treatment of blood products was introduced in 1985, the pattern of infection has changed. WHO figures (WHO–EC 1991) show that vertical or perinatal infection is the major route by which children acquire the virus; this now accounts for 70–80 per cent of HIV. The prevalence in children reflects the rising prevalence in women. Data from unlinked anonymous testing programmes of the newborn in inner London in 1991 showed a prevalence of 1 in 500; a fourfold increase in two years (Ades *et al.* 1991). More recently the use of zidovudine in pregnancy has been shown to reduce mother-to-baby transmission by two thirds (ACTG trial 1994).

THE CLINICAL PICTURE OF HIV INFECTION IN CHILDREN

Paediatric HIV and AIDS is a field with rapidly changing knowledge and with a range of complicated clinical problems. There have been improvements in the early diagnosis of HIV in babies and viral testing is now available in most paediatric centres in the UK. In adults viral load has been correlated with future disease progression but in children this is still unknown. However, it is very useful in following the response to anti-retroviral therapy. The natural history in children differs from that of adults. Approximately 20 per cent of children with vertically-acquired HIV infection develop severe disease in the first year of life. The remainder have a more slowly progressive course and the progression to AIDS is much slower (European Collaborative Study 1991). Data from the French and European Collaborative Study suggest that 40 per cent of children had AIDS by their fifth birthday and 25 per cent had died (Blanche *et al.* 1997).

Children with HIV infection may develop a wide spectrum of signs and symptoms, including opportunistic infections, encephalopathy, failure to thrive, recurrent bacterial infections, malignancy, and LIP. Most infected children have a number of coexisting illnesses and may be receiving treatment for acute infections at the same time as prophylaxis and treatment for persistent infections. They may also need symptom control. Treatment needs to be flexible through the different phases of the illness, with the emphasis on acute intervention and palliative measures changing as the disease progresses. It may be difficult to find a balance between making an overall plan for palliation and support focusing on the quality of life, and pursuing active intervention to increase life expectancy, and hoping that research may find a cure. Much will depend on the individual clinical situation as well as the family's wishes. The right of the child to consent, or not, to treatment and medical procedures, according to the principles of the Children Act 1989 must also be considered.

Some specific infections in symptomatic children

Some of the infections that carers may be less familiar with are detailed below. Much that is known is derived from the observation and treatment of adults with HIV and AIDS. It is likely that with increasing use of prophylaxis and the continued new developments in therapy survival is likely to improve in the future.

Pneumocystis carinii pneumonia (PCP)

This is caused by a commonly found protozoan, and carried by people and domestic animals. It is the most frequently reported opportunistic infection in children in Europe and the USA and has a high mortality. Definitive diagnosis is made by finding the organism on microscopy (through bronchoscopy with bronchio-alveolar lavage or lung biopsy). Treatment is generally with high-dose co-trimoxazole. Because PCP may be the first presenting illness associated with AIDS, primary prophylaxis (co-trimoxazole, three times weekly) is generally given to HIV positive children (Centre for Disease Control 1991; Hughes 1991).

Mycobacterium avium-intracellulare infection (MAI)

Before AIDS, MAI was rarely seen. It is still uncommon and generally a late complication. It has a non-specific presentation with recurrent fever, chills, abdominal pain, failure to gain or maintain weight, and diarrhoea. The outcome is generally poor. Treatment is usually with antituberculosis medication, however, some of the drugs commonly cause nausea and vomiting. Treatment decisions should be based on the child's general condition. Comfort and nutrition are the main issues to consider (Hanger and Powell 1990).

Cryptosporidiosis

Cryptosporidium is an enteric protozoan that can cause acute self-limiting disease in immunocompetent children, but severe and persistent enteritis in children with AIDS. Symptoms include fever, frequent and voluminous diarrhoea, weight loss, dehydration, nausea, and vomiting. A large number of drugs have been used but none with any great success. Diarrhoea should be controlled as far as possible with oral rehydration, antidiarrhoeal and anti-emetic drugs such as loperamide combined with codeine phosphate or opioids, if necessary. It may not be possible to prevent the diarrhoea but only to reduce the frequency to one or two times daily. It is becoming more common to give total parenteral nutrition through a central line, which can be decreased or stopped once the child is able to eat and the weight loss is controlled. In the terminal stages of the illness, care focuses on comfort and care, and invasive procedures and aggressive management are not appropriate.

Encephalopathy

Encephalopathy in children is usually due to HIV itself rather than to opportunistic infections. The reported prevalence is higher in the USA (50–90 per cent) than in Europe (20–30 per cent) (Belman *et al*. 1988). The European Collaborative Study (1990) has reported abnormalities only after the development of other severe manifestations. This geographic variation may be due to differences in patient recruitment in studies, as well as to the use of cocaine in mothers of infected children in the USA.

Encephalopathy may be static or progressive with the loss of developmental milestones, deterioration of motor skills in toddlers, and intellectual abilities and behavioural abnormalities in older children. Ataxia, pseudobulbar palsy, and acquired microcephaly may also occur. The only treatment is support and symptom management. Computed tomography (CT) or magnetic resonance imaging (MRI) scans may show cerebral atrophy or calcification, and will help exclude causes such as cerebral lymphomas or infections which might be treated aggressively.

THE UNPREDICTABLE COURSE OF AIDS

Families experience great uncertainty and a rollercoaster of emotions because of the nature of HIV and AIDS. The onset and presentation of the illness is variable and is followed by periods of illness and good health. Children may be symptom-free for an unpredictable length of time. Developmental delay and regression can be anticipated but not predicted. The child may be dying, then improve, and go on to live for weeks, months, or even years. Parents may have to go through anticipatory mourning and come to accept the loss, only to have the child recover leaving the family bewildered. This is further complicated by the important belief that you can 'survive and thrive' with AIDS.

Families must live with hope if they are to counter the overwhelming negative attitude of the media.

The unpredictable nature of AIDS can also lead to problems for staff. It is difficult to define a terminal phase clearly, which means for each exacerbation of the disease, a balance must be found between active intervention and facing the possibility that death is imminent. Sometimes it is possible to make a decision that death is indeed inevitable but at other times it is difficult to be sure. This compounds the problem for both family and carers, of being able to 'let go' and allow a child, for whom they have fought so hard, to die in peace.

After a child dies

The Advisory Committee on Dangerous Pathogens (1990) has offered guidelines for handling someone who has died of an AIDS related illness, but there is no doubt that for most people adoption of these guidelines will cause distress. They should be interpreted as sympathetically as possibly, as a caring and sensitive approach will help and support parents whose child has died.

As in life, care should be taken to avoid exposure to blood and other body fluids. Leaking wounds should be sealed with a waterproof, occlusive dressing. The body can then be laid out according to the family's wishes. It is then placed in a body bag and the body and bag labelled 'danger of infection'. Baby and child sized body bags are available.

It should be possible to prepare parents and to explain that, because of HIV infection, there may be certain restrictions about embalming and viewing the body after it has left the ward or their home. Some funeral directors will facilitate further opportunities for the family to see the child's body.

HIV and AIDS as a family disease

A young child may be the first member of a family to present with signs or symptoms which may be due to HIV infection. The issue of testing the child then broadens to include, by implication, also testing the mother and other family members. As well as facing the diagnosis of a life-threatening illness in their child, parents may simultaneously have to face the same diagnosis in themselves and their other children.

During the course of the disease, any family member may be ill, dying, or bereaved simultaneously. Often they will be at different stages of coping with their own illness and bereavement. This can leave them feeling alone, lead to conflicts of denial and acceptance, and make it difficult for family members to support each other.

The fear and stigma surrounding HIV and AIDS may lead parents to lie to family, friends, and neighbours, and to themselves, denying that the illness is due to HIV infection.

Consequences of this may include isolation, lack of support and sympathy, and guilt if the child dies. Depression and suicide may be a response to familial and social isolation, to guilt at having infected family members, to the perceived hopelessness of the situation, to the actual debilitation of the illness, or to the loss of an important relationship. Parents may feel there is nothing to live for, except to become symptomatic and join their children in death. Parents may sustain lies about the diagnosis even years after a child's death and isolation, unresolved mourning, and pathological grief are common.

In times of parental illness or death, practical issues about caring for the child emerge. It is preferable for the child to have consistent care, sustained over time, so that he or she does not have even more losses to cope with. In some communities the extended family or community will care for the orphaned children. Grandparents may also wish to care for their infected grandchildren, their own children having died. However, other families will depend on the statutory or voluntary facilities to provide care in these circumstances.

Helping the families

Every family has strengths, and by building on these strengths and providing respite and relief, families can be helped to live with HIV and AIDS. Power needs to be given to them to choose the type of care and support they want, and from whom they want it. Help can be given so they can focus on their strengths and resources and not just see their vulnerability and overwhelming difficulties (Bor *et al.* 1992).

A multidisciplinary approach to provide physical, social, spiritual, and educational support is ideal (Claxton and Harrison 1991). There needs to be good liaison between specialists and district general hospitals, and also between the hospital and the community. Without co-ordination, services can easily be duplicated while other needs may go unmet.

At the moment, most children are treated in specialist centres, predominantly in London. In addition to having related diagnostic capabilities and treatment options, they have staff who are specially trained and experienced with the unique complications and social problems seen in children with AIDS. However, a specialist centre may be unable to meet local needs, and it is likely that the majority of children will need both community and hospital based services. In some areas, there are home-care teams but these deal mainly with adults with HIV/AIDS and may have little or no experience nursing children. In each situation a team, which can work together to offer the family the help that it needs, must be built up using the expertise of the hospital, community paediatric nurses, palliative care teams, and the primary health-care team. Some specialist schemes also exist and may be helpful. Barnardos have established 'Positive Options' to help families with future child-care plans and they may be able to help parents negotiate with the authorities. Brenda House, in Edinburgh, for drug-using women, provides residential care for whole families. The different models of care are still developing and a variety of these may be called on as the families' needs for services change and increase over time.

During the illness, regular visits to hospital can provide a sense of purpose. For many, the hospital is a very real part of their lives. Parents get tremendous support from the staff, other parents, and parents support groups, who also seem to validate the importance of the child's life.

We can help by trying to normalize HIV and AIDS, restoring the family to problem-solving and coping abilities.

AIDS may require a shift in the structure of a couple's relationship and changes in role definition. Carers must also address the needs of the siblings. Parents can be helped by practical suggestions; videos, scrap-books, or memory boxes can be made and left with messages and mementoes for the surviving members of the family. There are voluntary organizations which can provide family support, feelings of acceptance, belonging, and information. Others offer spiritual support, and information about sympathetic ministers of different faiths is also available. (See Appendix B.)

As the disease progresses, there may be a time when no further aggressive treatment is possible, or it has been decided against. This means parents may have the opportunity to choose whether they wish to care for the child in hospital, in a hospice, or at home. Sometimes, there is no such clearly-defined terminal phase but the aim, wherever the child is cared for, needs to be based on the hospice philosophy and involve a partnership between the child, the family, and the care providers.

Conclusion

No one form of support, when used alone, can be effective in helping families cope with all the losses that living with HIV and AIDS brings. A combination of efforts works best, offering the family multiple choices and allowing them to discover what helps them the most.

REFERENCES

Ades, A. E., Parker, S., Holland, F. J., Davison, C. F., Cubitt, D., Hjelm, M., Wilcox, A. H., Hudson, C. N., Briggs, M., Tedder, R. S., and Peckham, C. S. (1991). Prevalence of maternal HIV-1 infection in Thames regions: results from anonymous unlinked neonatal testing. *Lancet*, **337**, 1562–4.

Advisory Committee on Dangerous Pathogens (1990). *HIV—the causative agent of AIDS and related conditions*, (2nd edn). HMSO, London.

Belman, A. L., Diamond, G., Dickson, D., Horoupian, D., Lantos, G., Llena, J. et al. (1988). Paediatric acquired immune deficiency syndrome. *American Journal of Diseases of Children*, **142**, 29–35.

Blanche, S., Tardieu, M., et al. (1990). Longitudinal study of 94 symptomatic infants with perinatally acquired human immunodeficiency virus infection. *American Journal of Diseases of Children*, **144**, 1210–15.

Blanche, S., Newell, M. L. et al. (1997). Morbidity and mortality in European Children vertically infected by HIV I. *Journal AIDS*, **14**, 298–302.

Bor, R., Miller, R., and Goldman, E. (1992). *Theory and practice of HIV counselling: a systemic approach*. Cassell, London.

Centre for Disease Control (1991). Guidelines for prophylaxis against *Pneumocystis carinii* pneumonia for children infected with human immunodeficiency virus. *Journal of American Medical Association*, **265**, 1637–44.

Chin, J. (1990). Current and future dimensions of the HIV/AIDS pandemic in women and children. *Lancet*, **336**, 221–4.

Claxton, R. and Harrison, T. (1991). *Caring for children with HIV and AIDS*. Edward Arnold, London.

Connor, E. M., Sperling, R. S. et al. (1994). Reduction of maternal–infant transmission of human immunodeficiency virus type 1 with zidovudine treatment. Paediatric AIDS Clinical Trial Group Protocol 076 Study Group. *New England Journal of Medicine*, **331**, 1173–80.

European Collaborative Study (1991). Children born to women with HIV-1 infection; natural history and risk of transmission. *Lancet*, **337**, 253–60.

European Collaborative Study (1990). Neurological signs in young children with HIV infection. *Pediatric Infectious Disease Journal*, **9**, 402–6.

Gibb, D. M., Duggan, C., and Lwin, R. (1991). The family and HIV. *Genito-urinary Medicine*, **67**, 363–6.

Hanger, S. B. and Powell, K. R. (1990). Infectious implications in children with HIV infection. *Pediatric Infectious Disease Journal*, **19**, 421–36.

Hughes, W. T. (1991). *Pneumocystis carinii* pneumonia: new approaches to diagnosis, treatment and prevention. *Pediatric Infectious Disease Journal*, **10**, 391–9.

WHO–EC Collaborating Centre on AIDS (1991). *AIDS surveillance in Europe*. WHO, Paris. Quarterly report no. 30, 29.

3
Symptom management

Ann Goldman and Roger Burne

When a child's illness is acknowledged to be incurable and the focus of care is palliative, it is often more helpful to concentrate on the individual child and his symptoms at the time, than look to textbook descriptions of the original diagnosis. Previous chapters have considered some of the different life-threatening illnesses and the particular problems they present. In this chapter, the management of the individual symptoms is considered in more detail, but drug doses are given in Appendix A.

Many children will have multiple problems; time and careful consideration should be given to each one individually. At first, only a very general and sometimes misleading idea of the real problems may be apparent; with careful evaluation the complexities of the problems will become more clear. Symptoms may be related to the disease itself, the treatment, or to unrelated illness. It is important to try and distinguish which are truly problems for the child, which for the family, and which are mainly for the professional helpers. When problems have been identified and assessed, a plan of management can be made. Once treatment begins, continuous evaluation is important so adjustments of the help being offered can be made as the situation changes.

ADMINISTRATION OF DRUGS

Children with chronic illness may be very good at taking regular medication. On the other hand, the illness itself may make it difficult or they may be extremely fed up with treatment. Thought needs to be given to arranging a regimen that will be most acceptable to the child and practical for the family. Sometimes, as a child becomes more sick, complex regimens are no longer possible and priority needs to be given to the most important medications.

Usually, oral medication is the route of choice. Some drugs may be given as liquids but children are often more willing and able to take tablets (whole or crushed) than we expect. If a child is no longer able to take drugs orally, for example as their level of consciousness decreases or if they are unable to swallow or have severe vomiting, another route must be used. Rectal administration is possible for many drugs and is acceptable for some children, although repeated use may lead to soreness. Many of the drugs used in palliative care can be given effectively subcutaneously. A simple syringe pump provides constant levels, is easy to establish and can be managed by parents. If the child already has an indwelling intravenous catheter, then this can be used, but it is rarely necessary to set up intravenous lines for terminal care.

PAIN

Pain is a complex sensation influenced not only by the degree of physical damage to the tissues but also by the psychological, social, and cultural factors which are unique to each person. Although this can make management difficult it also suggests the possibility of improving the pain by combining a number of different treatment approaches. Although pain is one of the problems most feared by the parent of a dying child, it is usual to be able to improve it very significantly. A small group of patients, however, including those with neuropathic pain, may be more difficult to manage. An important principle to keep in mind is not to ignore a child's complaint of pain. If in doubt, it is preferable to overestimate rather than undertreat it.

Assessment

It is essential to have as clear and as wide ranging an assessment of the pain as possible before developing a plan of management (Table 3.1). With children, their range of development, understanding, and communication skills can make this more difficult, and in the past this has contributed to neglect of pain in children. Nevertheless, a great deal can be learned from a systematic history from the child, with the parents' help. All the sites of pain should be considered and for each one, the details of nature, severity, time course, and influencing factors. Identifying individual painful areas is important as the causes of the pain, and therefore approaches to treatment, may be different for each. Often the use of a body outline completed in collaboration with the child and parent can be helpful (Fig. 3.1). A range of specific pain assessment tools for children have been developed in recent years. These can be used alongside history and examination, and can be particularly helpful when judging the value of treatments. The choice of which tool to use depends on the

Table 3.1   Assessment of long term pain

The pain itself:
• site
• nature
• severity
• timing
• precipitating and relieving factors

The child and family:
• coping skills
• past experience of pain
• anxiety and emotional distress
• meaning of pain

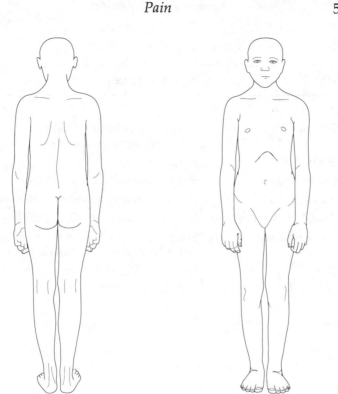

Fig. 3.1

child's development and the situation (Table 3.2). Assessment in the child with developmental delay and communication difficulties is particularly challenging and still depends on parental and staff observation.

Treatment

Individual or combinations of treatment can be chosen from a range of approaches (Table 3.3). Realistic goals for pain relief should be established with the child and family. Regular and frequent reassessment will then be needed to see if the goals are being achieved and to adjust the treatment accordingly.

Table 3.2 Tools for pain assessment in children

Method	Pain assessment
Self-report	
Description	Simple, depend on child's communication skills
Body chart	Wide age range
Colour scale	Simple intensity rating added to chart
Faces scales	Intensity rating for young children
Visual analogue scales	Intensity rating for older children
Numerical scales	Simple but intervals along scale may not be equal from child's perspective
Diary	Use of rating scale over time may reveal patterns of pain.
Behavioural	
Gauvain–Piquard rating scale	Relatively new, designed for longer term pain

Analgesic drugs

Drug therapy is the mainstay of analgesia for most terminally ill children. When a child presents with pain, it is usual to progress through a sequence of oral analgesics of increasing strength until the pain is relieved. However, if a child presents with severe pain, perhaps of sudden onset or because it has been neglected so far, stronger drugs should be used immediately and, if necessary, by other routes to provide rapid onset of relief. Analgesia should be given regularly to avoid pain recurring as drug levels fall, and to reduce the anxiety which 'waiting for pain' provokes.

The mild non-opioid analgesic of choice in children is paracetamol. This acts peripherally and is effective for mild to moderate pain, without side-effects. Paracetamol has a ceiling of efficacy so when pain is no longer relieved a mild opioid drug such as codeine or dihydrocodeine can be introduced. Potential side-effects of mild opioids are similar

Table 3.3   Approaches to pain management

Pharmacological
  Analgesics   mild
                    moderate
                    strong
  Non-steroidal anti-inflammatory agents
  Antidepressants and anticonvulsants
  Antispasmodics

Physical
  Radiotherapy
  Anaesthetic blocks
  Transcutaneous electrical nerve stimulators (TENS), acupuncture
  Massage
  Warmth, cold

Psychological
  Explanation, reassurance
  Distraction
  Hypnosis

---

to the stronger opioids and are described below. The main
clinical problem to anticipate is constipation. They also have
a ceiling analgesic level and if the pain is not helped, then
a stronger opioid should be considered. Morphine and
diamorphine are the drugs of first choice, as they have no
ceiling analgesic level and experience has not shown any
advantage in other preparations.

Many myths still remain for both the public and professionals about the use of strong opioids in children. Often,
good pain relief depends on tackling these myths and
enabling parents and carers to have the confidence to use the
strong opioid drugs appropriately. For parents, the use of
morphine may represent a final step in acknowledging that
their child's illness is terminal and, if so, this must be
addressed with them. They may fear that if you begin morphine now 'nothing will be left' if the pain increases later.
The lack of an analgesic ceiling with morphine should
reassure them. Parents and staff may have concerns about

addiction, but again they can be reassured. There is no evidence that psychological addiction occurs in patients treated with opioids for severe pain. Physiological tolerance will develop but if the pain resolves, for example after radiation to a bony metastasis, morphine can be withdrawn easily by gradually decreasing the doses to avoid symptoms of physical withdrawal. Professionals may be concerned about potential respiratory depression but there appears to be a wide margin between doses required for analgesia and those causing respiratory failure, with pain acting as a physiological antagonist to the respiratory depressant effects of morphine.

The route of choice for strong opioids is oral, as a liquid, or tablets which can be taken whole or crushed, or via a naso-gastric tube. A choice can be made between four-hourly or slow release preparations. Twice-daily medication with slow release morphine (MST) is a great advantage for children and convenient for home use. A starting dose can be estimated according to the child's weight but it then needs to be increased as necessary, to provide optimum analgesia and as the disease progresses. Some practitioners prefer to use a short-acting preparation initially and then change to slow release when a stable analgesic dose is reached. It is essential to also provide a short-acting preparation to use for break-through pain.

If the child is unable to take drugs orally (e.g. inability to swallow, vomiting, or decreased level of consciousness) other routes can be used. Some children are comfortable with rectal drugs and this route can be useful, especially in the last hours. Morphine suppositories (four-hourly) or MST tablets can be used. Otherwise a subcutaneous infusion of diamorphine is a simple and effective choice. They are easy to set up, well tolerated, and parents can be shown how to draw up and reload the syringes themselves. If a child already has established intravenous access then this can also be used.

Although a large number of side-effects of opioid drugs are known, in clinical practice, constipation is the main problem. Most children require regular laxatives and careful observation to avoid problems of constipation. Nausea and vomiting are rarely problems and prophylactic anti-emetics are not necessary. Many children are drowsy when they first start strong opioids and this should be anticipated so that parents do not become alarmed and think that the disease has progressed rapidly. Drowsiness tends to wear off after a couple of days. Some children experience itching which usually wears off, if not, antihistamines help, though occasionally it can be troublesome. Euphoria is rare but some children experience vivid dreams.

Reduced starting doses of strong opioids should be given to babies under six months old, as the side-effects are more common. Children with severe renal impairment must also be treated with caution; their dose should be built up gradually from a quarter to a half of the usual estimate and subsequent doses may be needed less frequently. Each patient's regimen will need to be worked out individually.

Co-analgesics

Other drugs may be helpful and can be used in combination with opioids. Non-steroidal anti-inflammatory agents are particularly helpful for bone and joint pain, or when there is an inflammatory component to the pain.

Nerve pain which characteristically has a stabbing, shooting, or burning nature tends to be much less responsive to opioids. Drugs which may help in this situation include low dose amitriptyline and anti-epileptic drugs such as carbamazepine. Steroids may also be useful to decrease swelling and inflammation at sites of nerve compression and tumour invasion.

Painful muscle spasms are a common problem in children with neurological problems and can be difficult to treat. Low dose diazepam is probably the most effective muscle relaxant. Drowsiness may occur but tends to decrease with time. Dantrolene and baclofen may be tried but response is variable. Sometimes spasm may be caused or worsened by pain and this should be treated. Regular gentle movement, hydrotherapy, and physiotherapy may also be helpful.

Cardiac pain resembling angina in nature, is sometimes a problem for boys with Duchenne's muscular dystrophy, and may be helped by glyceryl trinitrate taken by sucking tablets or via skin patches.

Physical approaches

For pain from a tumour, radiotherapy can be used palliatively as a potent analgesic if the tumour is accessible and radiosensitive. In recent years, the trend has been towards very short courses for pain relief and this is a great advantage to the child and family.

Anaesthetic blocks occasionally have a role if the pain has an appropriate distribution, for example the pain from a large liver tumour may be relieved by a coeliac plexus block. In children the widespread nature of their tumours at relapse means that blocks are rarely used. If a block is to be considered, the help of an experienced anaesthetist will be needed.

Other physical approaches such as the use of TENS (transcutaneous electrical nerve stimulators), massage, and warmth or cold may also be helpful.

Psychological approaches

Fear, anxiety, and boredom undoubtedly can make pain worse. It is important to give children an opportunity to talk about their pain, what it means to them, and any other fears and anxieties they may have. It is also important to maintain their interests and activities as much as possible both day-to-day and by providing realistic short-term goals. It is good to include the children themselves in the plans to manage their pain as the sense of control can be very helpful.

Hypnosis, distraction, and relaxation techniques often used to help with painful procedures also have a role in the pain of progressive disease. Children are often good subjects, they enjoy using their imagination and there are no unpleasant side-effects. Both children and parents can rapidly learn the process themselves and again benefit from this increased sense of control. These techniques can be particularly useful for children who have intermittent episodes of increased pain where raising the overall level of analgesics may cause unacceptable drowsiness; they are also helpful with insomnia and anxiety. Some nursing and medical staff have experience with the techniques, as do many child psychologists.

GASTROINTESTINAL PROBLEMS

Food and drink

Eating, chewing, and sucking form an important part of every child's life. These activities provide pleasure, stimulation, comfort, and reassurance, as well as nutrition. The significance of the mouth and the uses to which it is put depend on the child's age and developmental level. Children who are brain damaged, ill, or disturbed may regress in their behaviour and rediscover patterns normally associated with younger children.

Sustaining a child through providing food and nourishment is at the heart of being a parent. It can be very difficult to separate food from love and for some parents failing to be able to feed their child can equate on an emotional level with failing as a parent. For some ill people, one of the few activities over which they can retain any control will be their eating habits and this can lead to conflict during a chronic illness. If a parent is unable to persuade their child to eat, this becomes yet one more area of their child's life in which they no longer have any control.

Attitudes to food and drink for children with fatal illnesses need to be adjusted in line with their prognosis and general condition. Every child should be encouraged and helped to maintain normal activities, including eating and drinking as long as possible but children close to death should not be expected to eat or drink if these activities cause pain or distress. While every normal method of care should be used to ensure a child's comfort and well-being, invasive methods should not be used to prolong the process or distress of dying.

As stated in the previous chapter, feeding and swallowing cause particular problems for children with neurodegenerative diseases. In general, frequent small meals will be preferred. Careful attention to temperature, consistency, and flavour are important. Hard or dry foods should be avoided and sometimes a purée is easier to swallow than a liquid. Solids should be cut into small bite-size pieces and may be moistened with gravy or sauce. Uncooked dairy foods tend to thicken mucus and may be best avoided.

The child's position and surroundings must be carefully arranged to accommodate their individual needs and preferences. The child's head should be stabilized with the chin slightly tilted downwards, and help to close the lips while chewing may be needed. The swallowing reflex can be helped by gently stroking the child's neck. The feeder should check that the last mouthful has been swallowed before giving another, and should avoid scooping food off the child's chin with a spoon. There are a wide range of cups, spoons, plates, and other aids or appliances which may be of assistance. Choice of the right aid may prolong a child's ability to feed independently or ease the difficulties of feeding the totally-dependent.

Tube feeding and gastrostomy

Tube feeding is often regarded as a distressing and invasive procedure. Although this may be true it can be well tolerated by many children provided that modern small-bore silk tubes are used. While a nasogastric tube will enable fluids, food, and drugs to be given, it will not alleviate the problems which may be caused by excess secretions and may make them worse. With improved surgical techniques a gastrostomy can easily be fashioned and may be considered with the family if tube feeding is likely to be necessary for more than a short time.

No firm rules exist about assisted feeding for a child with a life-threatening disease. Each child and each situation must be considered individually and in discussion with the family. Usually it is reserved for those cases where significant distress will be alleviated or where it will extend a child's useful or enjoyable life. It can be helpful to discuss the issues earlier rather than later so that a considered policy may evolve gradually over a period of time.

For some children with slowly progressive diseases, when feeding becomes impossible but death is clearly not imminent, tube feeding or gastrostomy may be entirely appropriate. Sometimes a child might have had tube feeding instituted at an early stage of their disease, for example to maintain blood sugar levels in a metabolic disorder, and discontinuing it at a later stage would be more distressing for the family than maintaining it. In other situations, such as a child dying from metastatic malignancy, suddenly initiating tube feeding at a late stage in the disease would seem inappropriate and invasive.

Anorexia and dehydration

It is natural for those near to death to become less interested in food. Severely ill children, undertaking minimal activities, may survive extended periods of time in comfort, with surprisingly little nutrition. Failure to eat is often a problem for the family but not for the patient. Some reversible causes which should be considered are nausea, fear of vomiting, constipation, sore mouth, depression, or the presentation of too much or unappetizing food. If none of these are present, help should be focused on the family, helping them to acknowledge anorexia as part of the child's progressing disease. In adult palliative care, steroids are commonly used as an appetite stimulant. They are not recommended in children as they frequently result in unpleasant mood changes in the child and the rapid onset of a cushingoid appearance which the families and children themselves find disturbing.

Failure to maintain an adequate oral fluid intake tends to occur at a very late stage. In normal circumstances this would require urgent action but this, almost automatic, response can be inappropriate in a dying child. There is a widespread belief that dehydration is of itself distressing or uncomfortable, but experience in both the adult and paediatric hospice movements suggests that this is not so. Dehydration may even benefit some symptoms; vomiting and excess secretions are less likely, cerebral oedema is reduced, and as urine will be passed much less often, incontinence is reduced. The main discomfort of dehydration is a dry mouth, which can be helped by mouth care and moistening.

Mouth care

General debility and lowered immunity frequently lead to mouth problems in terminally ill children and, although they may be reluctant, regular mouth care is important. *Candida* infection is common and should be looked for regularly and treated with nystatin or ketoconazole. Mouthwashes or gentle cleaning and moistening using a foam stick with povidone-iodine 1% (Betadine), chlorhexidine gluconate 0.2% (Corsodyl), or hexetidine 0.1% (Oraldene) are useful, glycerine and lemon swabs are also available and attention to teeth will help. Sucking tinned unsweetened pineapple pieces, containing the proteolytic enzyme ananase, may also help. For painful ulceration or inflammation, benzydamine hydrochloride (Difflam) mouthwash has an analgesic and anti-inflammatory action. Benzocaine lozenges are numbing and may relieve pain. Choline salicylate gel (Bonjela) is also helpful but stings on first taking it. The range of tastes and sensations varies and personal preference is important. Dry lips are common and vaseline helps.

Nausea and vomiting

Vomiting is co-ordinated by the vomiting centre in the reticular formation of the medulla. It is induced by stimulation from the chemoreceptor trigger zone in the fourth ventricle, stimuli from the gastrointestinal tract, the middle ear, or higher centres. Anti-emetic drugs may work at one or a number of these sites (Fig. 3.2). Rationally they should be chosen according to the presumed cause of vomiting and often this approach is successful (Table 3.4). However, if vomiting is resistant then drugs which work at different sites can be tried and combinations active in different ways used together.

If possible, drugs can be given orally but if necessary rectal or subcutaneous routes can be used. A number of anti-emetics are compatible with opioids in a syringe pump and are not irritant when given subcutaneously. Cyclizine and haloperidol are the drugs of choice in this situation, metoclopramide can also be used. Methotrimeprazine which is

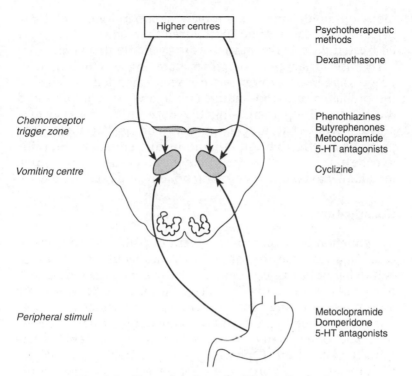

Fig. 3.2 Sites of action of anti-emetic drugs.

Table 3.4 Choice of anti-emetics

Opioids, uraemia, hypercalcaemia	Prochlorperazine, haloperidol, 5-HT antagonists
Gastric compression/stasis	Metoclopramide, domperidone
Bowel obstruction	Cyclizine, haloperidol, *not metoclopramide*
Raised intracranial pressure	Cyclizine steroids (if short-term), intrathecal methotrexate (for CNS leukaemia)

a strong sedative as well as anti-emetic can be chosen when sedation is also required. Prochlorperazine should be avoided as it is a skin irritant. Dystonic reactions with

metaclopramide and occasionally domperidone and haloperidol occur more often in children than adults. They may
be treated with benztropine or procyclidine if severe.

The use of steroids to reduce vomiting in children with
progressive brain tumours is not recommended, because of
the problems of mood changes, excessive weight gain, and
the need to keep increasing the dose as the disease progresses over what may be many months. Cyclizine is a
particularly effective anti-emetic in this situation. Steroids
may be a useful short-term emergency measure, for example
for a family to take with them on holiday and hold in reserve.

Constipation

Constipation is a common problem in palliative care. It can
cause anorexia, nausea, discomfort, and overflow diarrhoea.
A number of factors can contribute towards it, including lack
of mobility, poor or low fibre diet, low fluid intake, weakness
and muscle wasting, and some drugs, particularly opiates,
but also phenothiazines and anticholinergic drugs. At least
one, and often many of these factors are present in terminally ill children. If possible, it is preferable to anticipate
the problem by keeping note of bowel actions so that simple
measures and mild laxatives can be instituted quickly.
Constipation can be expected in almost all children taking
strong opioids, and laxatives should be prescribed regularly
at the same time.

Simple measures to combat constipation include increasing
a child's mobility if possible and improving their diet and
fluid intake. When laxatives are needed they can be chosen
from a range of drugs acting in different ways. Lactulose,
which is an osmotic laxative, retaining fluid in the bowel
and working over about 48 hours, is often well tolerated by
children but can be difficult to swallow by those with neurodegenerative disease. Stimulant laxatives act more quickly
and powerfully, by increasing intestinal motility but can also
cause abdominal cramp. Senna and bisocodyl are often
used, and co-danthramer, which is recommended only in
terminally ill patients, is used widely in adult hospice
practice.

Dioctyl (docusate sodium) has both stimulant and stool softening properties and is a good choice in children with painful fissures. If oral agents alone or combined, and in adequate doses, are unsuccessful, rectal preparations, either suppositories, such as bisocodyl, or enemas (Micralax, sodium citrate or enemette, docusate sodium) are almost always successful.

Diarrhoea

Chronic diarrhoea can be a problem for some children and can be very severe in some children with HIV infection. Loperamide given orally is usually effective but occasionally oral morphine is needed. If the diarrhoea is so severe that absorption of oral drugs is prevented, a subcutaneous infusion can be used.

Ascites

Children with progressive liver disease commonly develop ascites. Fluid restriction, spironolactone, and albumin infusions may help but paracentesis is only a very temporary measure.

Severe malignant ascites is uncommon in children. If unpleasant symptoms of abdominal distension, nausea, and vomiting from pressure on the stomach, dyspnoea, and leg oedema are present, treatment with diuretics (spironolactone and bumetanide) may help. Paracentesis may give good, but short-term symptom relief.

NEUROLOGICAL PROBLEMS

Convulsions

For some children, such as those with neurodegenerative diseases, seizures may have been a problem throughout their illness. For others, such as a child with metastatic malignancy, they may only develop terminally. Watching a child having a major convulsion can be extremely frightening particularly for parents caring for their child at home or if the fit was unexpected. It can be tempting for staff caring for a child who may, but is unlikely to have a fit, not to warn the parents, to avoid causing them unnecessary anxiety, but this is not recommended, as if the child has an unexpected fit the family will be much more distressed by being unprepared.

Children with known epilepsy will usually be on routine anticonvulsants. In general, these will be adjusted so that prolonged convulsions do not occur or are very rare. For some children, less than perfect control has to be balanced with drug side-effects, and parental wishes. A deterioration in the pattern of convulsions in a child with epilepsy can usually be approached by reviewing and altering the routine medication. In children with generally satisfactory control, but the occasional prolonged seizure, drugs for emergency use may be needed by parents but routine anticonvulsants may not need to be changed.

For emergency control of seizures, diazepam is an excellent drug but it needs to be used intravenously or rectally. Although it is good for terminating a fit, it does not have an extended anticonvulsant effect. Families caring for a child where fits are a possibility should have a supply of rectal diazepam available and be taught how to use it if necessary.

For continuing severe seizures, alternative drugs which can be used are midazolam, paraldehyde, or phenobarbitone. Midazolam is a benzodiazepine which can be given by continuous subcutaneous infusion and is both sedating and anticonvulsant. It is also compatible for infusion with opioids. Paraldehyde is painful when given intramuscularly but can be given rectally when diluted with an equal volume of arachis oil. Although traditionally it is given using a glass syringe, problems are unlikely using modern plastic syringes if it is given without delay. Phenobarbitone is not used routinely with childhood epilepsy because of its side-effects of sedation and behaviour problems, but these may not be applicable in the case of a terminally ill child, indeed sedation may be desirable. In the case of severe prolonged seizures it can be given subcutaneously through a syringe driver and the dose increased as necessary for control.

General supportive care to consider in a child having frequent or prolonged fits should include reducing fever, by the use of a fan, sponging, and paracetamol.

Anxiety and agitation

Drugs are not a substitute for time spent with a child listening to, and talking about their fears and anxiety, but they may nevertheless be useful in combination. Drugs may also be helpful when a child is very close to death when agitation and confusion may result from irreversible organ failure.

Benzodiazepines which are anxiolytic and sedative are often the first choice, either diazepam orally or midazolam via a syringe pump subcutaneously. Haloperidol which also has anti-emetic activity is useful and methotrimeprazine, a phenothiazine with anti-emetic and analgesic effects is a powerful sedative. Both of these can be given subcutaneously and are compatible with morphine.

SKIN PROBLEMS

Pressure sores

Fortunately, pressure sores are not a common problem in paediatrics but in children with prolonged illnesses and neurodegenerative conditions, the risk is increased. Many of the factors known to contribute to the development of pressure sores including lack of mobility, weight loss, incontinence, and poor nutrition may be present.

It is important to consider prevention. Encouraging mobility and frequent turning will help relieve pressure and friction but this must be balanced with the distress which may be caused from pain and other symptoms. There are also a number of aids designed specifically to help prevent pressure sores. Sheepskins, Spenco, and large cell ripple mattresses are readily available and easily managed at home. More expensive systems are rarely required.

If pressure sores have developed, the priority managing them in the dying child should be comfort and the prevention of complications. Occlusive dressings have the advantage of maintaining a low oxygen–liquid interface with the wound which decreases pain. These dressings do not need to be changed often (they last up to seven days), they can be removed easily, and healing is encouraged. Superficial sores can be covered with a semi-occlusive film (Opsite®) whilst on deeper sores, hydrocolloids (Granuflex®) are effective. Wounds that are very moist or infected can be covered with one of the alginate dressings (Sorbsan®, Kaltostat®).

Fungating tumours

Although these are rare in children, they are very distressing, especially if they are bleeding or smelly. Radiotherapy should be considered and occlusive dressings may reduce discomfort. Capillary oozing may be helped by topical 1 : 1000 adrenalin. Smell can be treated by reducing the anaerobic organisms, especially bacteroides, which colonize the ulcers. Topical metronidazole gel, available on special request, is very effective, and oral metronidazole or clindamycin will also help.

Itching

Many children with chronic debilitating illness suffer from dry skin and mild skin irritation. Simple measures such as avoiding soap and using oil in the bath, applying moisturizing cream and oils, wearing cotton clothes, and keeping cool can be suggested.

Generalized pruritus which can be severe may be associated with jaundice and cholestasis. Cholestyramine is the most useful medication and although it can be difficult for some children, many tolerate it surprisingly well. It can be taken with food or drinks like squash. Other drugs which may help are rifampicin and ursodeoxycholic acid.

Opioid drugs can cause histamine release and generalized itching, although it is not a common side-effect. It usually wears off or responds to an antihistamine such as chlorpheniramine, but occasionally is difficult to treat and may be helped by trying a different opioid preparation.

ANAEMIA AND BLEEDING

Anaemia

Chronic anaemia from poor dietary intake or in association with a chronic debilitating disease such as renal failure may have been a problem over many years. In children with progressive malignant disease, anaemia is often part of the terminal illness as the tumours involve bone marrow infiltration. Treatment at this stage of a child's life should be directed towards the symptoms of anaemia rather than the blood count and each situation must be judged at the time it occurs, and in consultation with the family. If the child's level of activity is very low the anaemia may cause very few symptoms. If the anaemia has developed more quickly and the symptoms of tiredness are interfering with what has otherwise been a good quality of life, red cell transfusions may be appropriate. This is often the situation in children with malignant disease. Families should be clear about the value and purpose of transfusions, and that there will come a point when the child's quality of life has declined to such an extent that they may no longer be appropriate. Transfusions of packed cells are usually done most conveniently in hospital as a day-case or overnight admission.

Bleeding

For a child to die from a massive bleed is frightening for the patient, distressing for the carers, and may leave the family with unforgettably painful memories of the time of death, so strong efforts should be directed to prevent the situation. If it is possible that an overwhelming haematemesis or haemoptysis might occur it is valuable to have an appropriate analgesic and sedative injection readily available, to relieve distress, such as diamorphine and methotrimeprazine.

Doses should be calculated and prescribed and the ampoules and syringes easily accessible either in hospital or at home.

Serious bleeding may be associated with portal hypertension and oesophageal varices in children with liver disease. Treatment for this has been helped in recent years by sclerosis of the varices with injections of ethanolamine, via an endoscope. Children with liver disease may also have low levels of clotting factors which may be helped by regular vitamin K and low platelets from hypersplenism.

Children with progressive malignancy, particularly leukaemias, also frequently have low platelets though serious bleeding is uncommon. Earlier in their illness, a child may have received platelet transfusion according to the platelet level (below 20×10^9/litre). During terminal care, routine platelet transfusion is not regular practice and is reserved for bleeding problems which interfere with the quality of life; persistent nose bleeds or haematemesis, for example but not just petechiae. However, children with acute promyelocytic leukaemia or who have had a strong history of significant bleeding problems may require regular platelet transfusions.

Platelets only take a short time to infuse and can be given readily at home, especially if the child has a central line *in situ*. Routine cover or immediate access to hydrocortisone and antihistamines should be available. Haemostatics such as tranexamic acid may help reduce spontaneous bleeding even when platelets are low. These can be taken as tablets or used as a mouthwash for bleeding gums and mucous membranes.

DYSPNOEA

Respiratory symptoms which may cause distress to children and anxiety and concern for parents include dyspnoea, cough, and excess secretions. Haemoptysis is fortunately rare but the possibility can be particularly frightening. The degree of distress often depends on the speed of onset of the problem and the patient's level of anxiety as well as the severity of the underlying disease.

Consider the cause

It is helpful to try to consider what is the underlying problem giving rise to any symptoms so that treatment can be directed to relieving it if possible, as well as managing the symptoms. As well as pulmonary disease, such as damage, infection, malignant infiltration or pleural effusion, respiratory distress can also result from cardiac failure, superior vena caval obstruction or extrathoracic problems such as anaemia, ascites, or chest-wall pain. Even though treatment directed at these, such as radiation or drainage of ascites or effusions, may only be temporary, the relief produced may be worthwhile and should be considered.

Treating the symptoms

If the underlying cause of dyspnoea is not amenable to treatment, then the best possible relief can be worked towards by combining a variety of drug methods with practical and supportive approaches. Fear is often a powerful element in respiratory distress. The confidence of the staff to manage the situation, including acute problems, conveys itself to families even without words. Simple practical measures should be chosen according to what seems to help each individual. Not crowding the patient, using a fan, keeping curtains and windows open, finding the optimum position with pillows or a table in front to lean on, and relaxation exercises may all help.

The sensation of breathlessness can be decreased with opioid drugs which are usually given orally, or if necessary subcutaneously. Recently, nebulized morphine, sometimes with lignocaine has been introduced for adult patients with malignant disease and this also appears to give good relief of dyspnoea. Opioids and nebulized local anaesthetic agents are also helpful for coughing, which can be distressing, by aggravating chest-wall and headache pain, and disturbing sleep. It is usually recommended that patients fast for two hours after nebulized local anaesthetic. Any element of reversible airways obstruction, especially in a child with a past history of asthma can be treated with bronchodilators or steroids. A small dose of a sedative such as diazepam is often helpful in relieving the anxiety associated with dyspnoea.

Excess secretions may be a chronic problem for children with neurodegenerative disease, as their disease progresses and they are less able to cough and swallow. This may also occur in other terminally ill children as they near death. The use of a portable sucker at home is often helpful for children with a chronic problem but less appropriate for those nearing death. Hyoscine hydrobromide can be used to reduce secretions. Scopaderm patches are a convenient and acceptable way to give it or it can be given subcutaneously and is compatible with diamorphine if a pump is being used.

Children who have had a chronic disease such as cystic fibrosis with gradually increasing hypoxaemia, may suffer from headaches, nausea, drowsiness in the day, and poor quality of sleep at night. Intermittent or eventually continuous oxygen may help relieve the symptoms and can be given at home via nasal prongs. Children with malignant disease with dyspnoea in the late stages of their illness do not usually find oxygen helpful and often dislike the use of facial masks or prongs. Haemoptysis occurs quite frequently as a complication of advanced cystic fibrosis but is uncommon with malignant disease. Fortunately it is usually only streaking and small clots of blood but occasionally a massive bleed may occur and be a terminal event (see p. 71).

COMPLEMENTARY THERAPIES

Many families whose children have life-threatening and life-limiting illnesses look to complementary therapies. As yet, there is no convincing evidence from trials that these forms of therapy can contribute to curing the illnesses. However, many families believe that their child's sense of well-being and suffering from symptoms have been helped. Many different alternative approaches are available and often the therapists are willing to work in conjunction with conventional medicine to provide the best possible care for the child; indeed some of the practitioners of homeopathy and acupuncture, in particular, are also qualified in conventional medicine. Unfortunately, occasionally, families become involved with less scrupulous therapists who make unrealistic claims, subject the children to inappropriate forms of treatment, and charge high prices. As in conventional therapy, the child's welfare should be the priority and guiding principle for all those involved in care.

FURTHER READING

Hain, R. D. W. (1997). Pain scales in children: a review. *Palliative Medicine*, **11**, 341–50.

Hilgard, J. R. and LeBaron, S. (1984). *Hypnotherapy of pain in children with cancer*. William Kaufman, Los Altos.

Oxford Textbook of Palliative Medicine, Doyle, D., Hanks, G., MacDonald, N. (1997). Second edition, Oxford University Press, Oxford.

Regnard, C. and Tempest, S. (1998). *A guide to symptom relief in advanced cancer*. Haigh & Hochland, Cheshire.

Royal College of Paediatrics and Child Health (1997). *Prevention and control of pain in children*. BMJ, London.

Schechter, N., Berde, C., and Yaster, M. (1993). *Pain in infants, children and adolescents*. Williams & Wilkins, Baltimore.

4

Support for the family

Avril Trapp

The three of us had a very intense relationship. We had a desperate need just to be in each other's presence. Time together was so precious and appreciated.

When it was inevitable that Peter would soon die we tried to make sure he lived right until the moment. The three of us were together and Peter died knowing how much we loved him. He seemed to have an insight. He was calm, peaceful, and trusting. We are the luckiest and proudest parents in the whole world.

This was written by Peter's mother when he died aged eight, after treatment failed to secure any long-term future for him. This family had made decisions together about how to manage Peter's death.

Every family has decisions to make, and every family handles death differently. Offering support often means helping family members to make informed choices about their needs and enabling them to feel secure with their decisions, in what can be an ever-changing situation. What is written in this chapter can only suggest possibilities. Sometimes options are very limited, and families must choose carefully what is important, feasible, and right for them, and make decisions which result in the least long-term damage to the rest of the family. Families need to be able to look back on their decisions comfortably.

In this chapter, I have given some thought to the family, which should include parents, siblings, and grandparents, and also to the wider community. Ideally we think of these people linked together, relieving and assisting each other's burdens and fears, with effective communication flowing back and forth, as a large extended network. However, the reality may be that though people live together and take from each other, often each person has to cope independently with their own emotions during the period of the child's terminal illness. In this chapter, too, is a consideration of our own attitudes and emotions when offering help to families. A literature review is not included as these are available elsewhere (Van Dongen-Melman and Sanders-Woudstra 1986, Cincotta 1993).

DISCOVERING THE FAMILY

Our effectiveness in working with a family may be determined by our initial approach, the relationship we form, and the understanding we develop. Who are this family? Who do they consist of? What do they value, need, demand, and fear? What are their dreams, now and for the future? The answers to these questions may never be clearly found, or indeed openly spoken about, and exploring them involves a process of sensitive discussion and searching. The picture develops in small pieces, like a jigsaw which cannot be bent or broken to fit.

At the beginning of this search to understand the family, there must be genuine interest and sincerity. We, as helpers, have no right to automatic acceptance by a family. Acceptance in its true sense is worked for, hard-earned, and very precious, but without it our contribution will be limited. Families and individuals assess, as we do ourselves, who they will give their time and trust to, and what they will say and not say, and why. We sometimes realize that the family we want to work with, will not choose to work with or invest in us; they may have made other commitments and might not have the energy or desire for any form of new involvement at this time. Families make choices in relationships and we must respect these. We must also accept working with the family relationships as they are, we are the newcomers.

Discovering the family also means learning about yourself in each situation, what you have to offer, what you can cope with and what are your limitations. You must consider whether your goals, aims, and expectations are realistic in each circumstance, and you must try to understand how much you can expect of yourself and others. What is your own role in each situation and what, if any, defences do you need to use to remain effective? It is important not to work in isolation but to share, consider, and discuss with colleagues who share your work with this family. Examine your communication with each family member and consider whether it is effective or necessary so you can target whom you can help and whom you cannot. You may need to consider who may be able to help those whom you cannot.

It is important to consider the effects on people's lives if you try to encourage change. Change must happen with agreement, respect, and understanding. Take an overview of how the whole family works and how communication between everyone takes place (Mastroyannopoulou 1997). If, for example, a family member temporarily chooses denial to help then through their difficulties, this may be the right course for them. Family functioning is a very individual matter; a pattern may have developed in certain ways for special reasons. Here are some of a wide range of patterns.

1. One parent may be less able to face stress and the thought of death than the other, and so may choose to avoid a situation where they are expected to accept responsibility for caring for an ill child.

2. One parent may have been treated as a child by their partner throughout the marriage, and when expected to be a supportive adult parent they may crumble.

3. Some parents may have always overprotected their children and now have to face the reality that over-protection is not meeting the needs of the child.

4. A child may have a very close relationship with one family member and exclude another. This can be very painful for the excluded one(s) or it may be something of a relief.

5. The child who is ill may have always had a poor relationship with his parents.

6. One partner may seek strength and advice from their parents or friends and be dependent on them. The spouse may hold a very secondary position.

7. The marriage may have been unsatisfactory before the illness of a child. Partners may be forced apart or drawn closer together.

Each family will have their own list of what they need from helpers, that is, what they see as important to keep them going, and functioning well. Most will never have had a dying child before but may have had experience of severe illness and/or long-term distress and uncertainty. Most families will have some hopes, fears and expectations of us as helpers. These expectations will vary for each family but may include some of the following:

• that we help family members to fulfil their own expectation of themselves and achieve what is important for them;
• that we will be consistent, honest and reliable and work in a helpful way;
• that we share, support, and work together without becoming an added pressure on the family;
• that we listen to what is and is not said;
• that we recognize that needs may be different for each family member;
• that we do not de-skill the family by coming into their home and diminishing their confidence;
• that we respect their right to privacy;
• that we offer them time to absorb what is happening; to be themselves and reject what is unimportant in their individual situation;
• that we help support their need to do things their way and resist pressure to act in ways which do not suit them;
• that we are available and accessible.

Not only do families vary, but we as workers and helpers are all different. Many of our past experiences affect how we cope with personal hurt and how much we are able to share our feelings. When helping families, we need to acknowledge that they see us and our flaws too and, usually, still accept us into their difficult situation.

This is the family's time. A time of great preciousness mixed with personal torment, the pain of anger and disbelief at what is happening. Sometimes, there is an urge to hide from reality, risking resultant isolation. There is often a need to withdraw; not to have to cope with other people's embarrassment and well-meaning but, perhaps, superficial sympathy. Often families are defiant against the world. Many are searching for a meaning and at the same time experiencing feelings of failure and dispair.

Families have to face the anger and guilt of knowing they will carry on living, coupled with the anger and anguish that their child is dying. They have to protect and encourage each other when they are uncertain and frightened themselves. Such is their confusion very often that the greatest help may be to remind them that the treatment team will accept and concentrate on what they themselves deem important.

PARENT OR PARENTS

Some principles to follow when working with families

- Listen to what the parents and child say.
- Observe their communication together.
- Be aware of feelings of guilt, anger, denial, self-deception, and grief.
- Help them express feelings.
- Pinpoint their fears.
- Encourage reality.
- Identify their hopes and expectations.
- Focus on their strengths.
- Ensure they have access to information.

Fears and feelings

In discussion, it is important to go at the family's pace but some areas almost inevitably need to be explored and may need to be raised by the helper. Parents frequently feel totally helpless and consider themselves poor parents if they 'can't even prevent their child dying'. They may fear they aren't normal and that they are going mad, that this situation is not really happening, and is all a terrible dream. They worry about whether they will be strong enough. Parents fear the course of events; what death will look like, whether they will recognize when it is happening, and what they should do when the time comes. They need information and practical details to help maintain their confidence and sense of control.

This can be a time of great contrasts. The parent may sometimes want his child to die, for it all to end, and yet at the same time say 'Oh, he's no bother, I can manage, just as long as he's alive'. At times self-deception is employed; for example 'as long as the situation continues, it is as though the illness is beaten'. At the same time the parent wonders 'How can I keep going? How will I be able to stop?'

Some parents have to cope with feeling guilty at not searching for experimental treatment or, conversely, at using it and witnessing the side-effects. Some families feel that they are the cause of the death, whether by some genetic link or some unthinking act, or simply by admitting that the child cannot be kept alive any longer.

Each parent may cope differently, leading to misunderstanding and a feeling of being unsupported by the partner. The whole family dynamic can change, with one parent spending much more time with the family than previously. A child may direct anger or withdrawal at one parent, or relationships can be cemented in a special way. Our goals in offering support will have to be tailored to what is realistic in each family, but can include encouraging them to meet each other's needs as far as they can. This may mean an agreement that they seek support elsewhere, because they cannot offer it to each other. This is very normal and allows energies to be recharged but can lead family members to feel they are failing one another.

Often parents fear that they will not know what to say if difficult topics are raised. It is important to know what they are comfortable with. There is often a tendency for parents to overprotect their child and the worker must avoid overprotecting the child and the parents in collusion.

One child said to me, 'This is our time to be close, help my mother see that I want to talk about this. She is hurting so much but is so busy with unimportant things, she prevents us being close.' Eventually she did allow herself to be very close to her child and stopped avoiding him, when she was able to realize that it was fear and desire to remain in control that was affecting her.

Alternatively, there are parents who cannot acknowledge their child's impending death because it is too painful. The children do not wish to upset them, and remain silent on the topic.

Parents are frightened of getting things wrong. They feel they only get one chance. Professionals are also frightened. We, like parents, want to get it right, which is a terrible strain for us all. It should be a partnership, acknowledging that we are all trying to make things as good as possible, according to an individual family's priorities.

Helping parents cope

Parents usually need honesty and time to be listened to, as does every member of the family, but they do not need over-optimism because they then feel let down as if the worker, too, cannot face the realities. Most parents have buried levels of pain, anger, emptiness, questioning, disbelief, reality, 'dreamlike' feelings, and sadness. The family members may need to be able to express blame and hurt yet know that people understand. It may be very upsetting because the child they have loved and known may have changed and 'disappeared from sight some time ago'. One family removed all the mirrors in their home to hide the truth from themselves and the child. Professionals have to try to be relaxed and not embarrassed by the families' expressions of needs.

Parents usually develop their own coping mechanisms. They can be encouraged and their ideas validated. They may want reassurance and confidence that they are good parents.

They can also be offered suggestions of what others have found helpful.

Emphasis may be in several areas, as listed below.

1. Giving time to what is important and living in the present. At first this may be week-to-week, or day-to-day, but later, when time is shorter, from hour-to-hour is enough.

2. Finding ways to share time and caring when it is exhausting. One parent may sleep late when the other is with the child. It may be helpful for parents to have respite periods, where trusted relatives, friends, or professionals can help, but not to feel things are being taken out of their hands.

3. Consideration of financial implications. Both partners may have been earning and they will still be living at the same level of financial commitments and may be losing their homes or having great difficulties just when they cannot give their attention to such matters. (See Chapter 7.)

4. Helping to give some time to their own needs. In a way, this may be a dilemma in itself because they may have forgotten who they really are, after what may be many years of meeting others' needs in hospital and at home. They will probably be very tired. Although together in trying to ease their child's death, they may have no energy for strengthening their marriage and giving much to each other at this time. It can bring together or tear apart. One partner may feel they can only cope by being at work constantly or spending all the time with the siblings.

5. Validation of parents' chosen coping strategies. Making decisions for a family is de-skilling and destructive. Parents need to acknowledge their own values and be comfortable looking back on their decisions after death.

As death approaches, and pain and symptoms are under control families often choose to withdraw to the space they have chosen. Often this is one room where they all sleep together or perhaps a settee in the living room. In the hospital, consideration needs to be given to creating such personal space.

There is then a special time when the outside world seems unimportant. During this time, the family may arrange to do things precious to them. Favourite music is played, stories told, words spoken, feelings expressed. Often photographs and letters are looked at, more videos may be taken and families relive events together. This is a time of preparation and sharing. It may be enough for the family to have a nurse or doctor on call whom they trust and who is able to help, and come in and out, over this period as needed.

The team approach is crucial. When parents observe good communication between professionals on their behalf, this adds to their feelings of security. The team should be very flexible in its approach. It is unlikely that you will be the only professional going into the home. You need to communicate and work together for the same ends.

Not everyone, of course, has this period of waiting and preparation. Sudden death in whatever form, makes it necessary for members of the team to find ways to help a family cope and take in the reality. Spending time with the dead child, talking about what has happened to their child, and saying to the child all the things they would have said during a more prolonged terminal period may help, as do photographs of the family holding their child together. Most people are frightened of things they have not experienced and for which they have had no preparation. The suddenness of some situations means you may meet with a family you have not known previously. An open mind during this period will help you to be a friend and comforter, and encourage them to find strength to see and absorb what they cannot avoid.

THE CHILD

The child who is dying needs to know that he is not excluded or isolated, that he can still be himself, be valued, be complete. The child also needs to be able to blame and hurt, and yet know that those who matter most to him will understand. He will want to be spoken to as an ordinary person, be able to depend upon a consistency of care and live within the usual boundaries that make things secure for him. The worker must not confuse his or her own needs with those of the child. It is important to try to discover the person, what they value, fear, speak about, leave unspoken and demand. Most children give signals that help us to understand and we should respect their wishes and choices (Fig. 4.1).

All this will be affected by the patterns of communication in the family; whether they are 'open' or 'closed', whether the child feels he or she will be listened to, and whether his/her choices are feasible and can be achieved. It will also be influenced by the parents' and child's attitudes. Often, children give leads which people cannot bear to acknowledge, and children then accept that their attempts to communicate may not be successful. When children realize they have no control over situations they may become sullen, diffident, and withdrawn.

Children are usually very perceptive; they realize when no more can be done in the form of treatment and it is often a relief to them. However, the parents' need for the child to survive, may mean the initiation of some form of treatment that very often results in more time in hospital. Occasionally

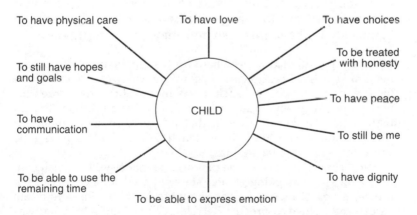

Fig. 4.1

a child may scream, protest, and withdraw personal consent and co-operation. Then the parents, family, and multi-disciplinary team lose the child not only physically, but in every other way.

One little five-year-old girl, Elizabeth who was greatly protected by her parents, screamed that half her body was dead and the other half was trying to follow.

Another six-year-old refused to speak to anyone and wanted merely to stop and go home. She died within a few days almost as though enough had been enough, as though she'd been let down by people continuing to fight something she'd chosen not to fight.

Learning to find the way to approach children equally, openly, and naturally is valuable. There can be a tendency to speak down to children because they unsteady you and make you feel insecure. Children will often take on the patterns expressed by their parents, as they realize it is easier for everyone. It is wrong for people to be over-optimistic; children who have been ill for a while will easily see through this and realize that the over-optimism is for their parents or the health worker. It is right to try to put things in perspective and encourage careful, meaningful use of time. Often the thing valued most is 'being normal'. Unfinished business and things of importance can be addressed by the child. This time can be so special in an open atmosphere but it must be accepted that this is not possible for everyone and to expect patterns to change totally in a home is unrealistic. Families who have never shared may continue this way.

Michael, aged 19, had worked hard for his university place. During his first year his illness recurred again; he was worried about how his friends would cope. He felt it was inappropriate to burden his new friends with what was happening to him and asked me to help them when he died to explain that he did care about them but conversation in the Students Union had appeared to have little space for what was facing him.

Mary, aged 17, was a single parent, a teenager with a small son. Realizing she was going to die, she prepared for her son in the future, a box of memories and thoughts for him. She wrote him letters and helped to prepare herself and her family for what was coming as well as setting down her wishes regarding legal custody.

BROTHERS AND SISTERS

To a large extent the needs of siblings are not very different from those of the patient; to be told what is happening, why it is happening, and as far as possible what is likely to happen in future. Excluding children from information seems to be unsuccessful in reducing their pain, as clearly they sense that something is seriously amiss and, in the absence of age-appropriate explanations, are prone to fantasize. (Lansdown and Goldman 1988; Pettle and Lansdown 1986).

Most brothers and sister have some difficulties. Many cope with a mixture of feelings and express frustration, anger, and fear about what is going to happen. They experience resentment that they may have to bear the brunt of their parents' constant changes in emotions. Sometimes they feel lonely, sad, isolated, unloved, and displaced. They may think they have lost their position in the family and feel second-best, believe they are in a no-win situation whatever they try to do. The sick child can resent the sibling at times and make his or her life more difficult and the sibling may be jealous of the sick child but find it difficult to express anger to people about their dying brother or sister. The sibling is also surrounded by uncertainty and by the fear of what is to come, the balance of their life is distorted. What might have been secure is now not, and boundaries are no longer fixed.

It is important that people close to the siblings such as friends and school teachers are aware of the strains and pressures they have to bear. Siblings often have to continue with the normal and extra pressures unaided, such as new school, exams, bullying, parents arguing, and being shunted around to different carers. Some siblings say that they feel they cannot share their feelings with their parents because they know their parents cannot cope with another thing and so they protect them. Schools can help by identifying one person to whom the sibling can go should there be difficulties. Alternatively, school can be their one place where things remain the same, and they are acknowledged for themselves. Some siblings survive by working very hard to achieve. Most siblings need a close friend outside of the family. Teenagers may feel very alone with their feelings and sometimes show signs of upset such as personality changes, aggressive, disruptive behaviour, sleeping disorders, nightmares, nervousness, being sad, anxious, and depressed.

Siblings are very important to each other (Davies 1991). They protect one another, older ones help to care for younger ones. They teach one another and share times of learning. They may come to each other's defence against parents in the form of sibling alliances. They confide in each other and share secrets from the rest of the world.

Siblings need to feel part of the process of their brother's and sister's death. They may have been their brother's or sister's closest confidant(e). They need to be able to speak about what they see happening, and to be reassured that what they feel is normal. They should be encouraged to do and say what is important to them as well as continuing some of the relationship they have always had. However, they, like everyone, will not talk to people who do not listen. Everyone needs someone they trust and it is hard to trust a person who does not tell you the truth. It is different in each household but sometimes families where communication is not open will be frightened that a sibling will share 'unacceptable' information with the sick child. The situation can be particularly difficult if the sick child is making the brother's and sister's lives a misery.

Being present at the death can be helpful when it is a calm and peaceful planned experience. Sharing feelings and emotions as a family, hugging, laughing, and crying together, acknowledging each other's needs on equal terms, though painful, can help for the future.

However, many parents may not realize, or have no energy left to acknowledge the importance of sibling involvement. They see themselves as protecting them from something too difficult and painful. To try and prevent difficulties later, it is important to help families to consider siblings' needs. They are part of the family and an important part of the life of the child who is dying. They should be helped to have the opportunity to share in and to be there at the death and have the opportunity to spend time with their brother's or sister's body so that they can say good-bye, and not be frightened of, or retain fantasies about, the unknown.

THE COMMUNITY

The child and his/her family have many contacts in the community. They encompass a wide range of people who may be involved during the child's illness (Fig. 4.2).

Professionals and friends need to be relaxed, unintrusive, supportive, and flexible. Everyone, the nurse who is helping with pain control, the local pharmacist, the neighbour who hands in a casserole, the parent network at hospital, clinic, school, or nursery, has a sensitive part to play in enabling people to feel cared for and loved.

One mum on her way to her son's funeral said that when the lollipop man stood with his head bowed, his cap in his hand at the school crossing when James's hearse went past, she felt both pride and gratitude yet it nearly broke her heart.

Schools and peers

Peers can be of great importance to children and fulfil various needs not met by others. Parents who overprotect their children may wrongly deny them these valuable oppor-tunities which help to keep the child in touch with the outside world, to be normal, and talk of normal things even though they may know that they are being left behind. Peers can offer the possibility of sharing thoughts on an equal basis without having to protect. Conversely, they can help dispel the natural pretence that it is not happening.

The headteacher and staff can be most helpful in enabling children to be at school, through having a flexible attitude as well as offering appropriate tuition, at home when necessary. A normal school environment where a child can compete and achieve even though he or she is dying, is most precious. If pupils and staff maintain involvement with the

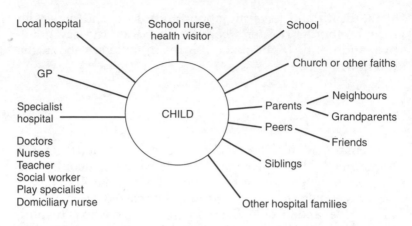

Fig. 4.2 The child and the family in the community.

child it helps to reduce isolation. Peers themselves may need to be helped to cope after the child's death and through the bereavement processes. They and the form-teacher may need to share and relive the experience together.

Grandparents

Grandparents can be a source of great strength or another pressure. It all depends on the person, their attitudes, and their relationship with their family. They bear a double grief—their grandchild's pain and their own child's pain. They are often in a difficult position receiving only little information, second-hand. Their advice may be sought, but then ignored and often their practical help is accepted but their own grief barely acknowledged. They may become very anxious, exhausted, feel helpless, or be domineering. Sometimes they are unable to cope and may try to shield the child and siblings. The advice they give may be based on over-protection, working against openness, and inhibiting the children and grandchildren from communicating freely. Most grandparents feel a terrible guilt that they will still be alive when their grandchild will be dead. This seems to be totally against the natural order of things and grandparents may feel especially powerless because of this.

Parents say it is extremely hard to feel close to the wider community. Things that were important before now do not matter. Values are different. Long-term planning becomes 'a day at a time'. Family members are not prepared to 'suffer fools gladly', are more direct and are unwilling to be put upon. The family feel anger at people who complain about seemingly minor things.

It is necessary to acknowledge that some people in the community say things inappropriately, that some people try to ignore what is happening, and that the media can on occasions distort facts and cause great distress. The majority of the time, however, everyone's efforts are acknowledged and appreciated.

CONCLUSION

Everyone in the family is affected by a child's death and everyone in the family needs to acknowledge the pain of parting. It is real and it is what we experience for loving each other.

Supporting families is a very special task and each family is different. Much of what you bring to this work will depend on your past experiences. Your relationship with a family is a partnership and within it you will offer different things to different members of a family enabling them to make choices, to act accordingly, and to feel comfortable with their own choices and actions.

All of us have our own experiences of bereavement, loss, or pain, which inform our work and which affect us in ways which we need to recognize and share. We can all feel the range of emotions that mirror those of the family members, anger, frustration, denial, exhaustion. We may reach a point of feeling empty and inadequate ourselves, and need to recognize the need to recharge our batteries.

Often we are left wondering where our responsibilities end and whether we will be able to cope. Very often we draw strength from the family itself, and most professionals can safely share their pain with their multidisciplinary team, who can recognize hurt and give support. Ultimately, like the family members we are all only human and the recognition of that fact, and the ability to respond in an open, honest way with the families with whom we work, may be our greatest strength.

REFERENCES

Cincotta, N. (1993). Psychosocial issues in the world of children with cancer. *Cancer* (supplement), **71**, 3251–60.

Davies, B. (1991). Responses of children to the death of a sibling. In *Children and death*, (ed. D. Papadoutou and C. Papadatos) pp. 125–33. Hemisphere, Philadelphia.

Lansdown, R. and Goldman, A. (1988). The psychological care of children with malignant disease. *Journal of Child Psychology and Psychiatry*, **29**, 556–67.

Mastroyannopoulou, K., Stallard, P., Lewis, M., and Lenton, S. (1997). The impact of childhood non-malignant life threatening illness on parents: gender differences and predictors of parental adjustment. *Journal of Child Psychology and Psychiatry*, **38**, 823–9.

Pettle, S. and Lansdown, R. (1986). Adjustment to the death of a sibling. *Archives of Disease in Childhood*, **61**, 278–83.

Van Dongen-Melman, J. E. W. and Sanders-Woudstra, J. A. R. (1986). Psychosocial aspects of childhood cancer; a review of the literature. *Journal of Child Psychology and Psychiatry*, **27**, 145–80.

5

Communicating with children

Richard Lansdown

Many parents and staff worry about what to tell a child about his or her illness, and whether and when to say that death is near. No rigid and simple answers exist to these questions, but it is valuable to know that evidence does suggest that those families who can express themselves openly benefit both during the child's illness and after the death (Spinetta *et al.* 1981). This chapter aims to give those working with dying children and their families, confidence and skills to encourage openness and to help reduce their anxiety and fears.

The consensus opinion in the literature has moved over the last 20 years from a protective approach to children towards honesty and openness (Chesler 1986). A number of factors have contributed to this shift. Direct observation of children with serious illness has demonstrated that many acquire considerable information about their disease, including the possibility of death, without being told specifically. This happened even to children who were cared for by staff and parents who believed that the children would remain naïve and protected if their disease was not discussed with them (Bluebond-Langner 1978, Kendrick *et al.* 1987). Frankness in communication is also in sympathy with society's changing expectations in health care. Patients and families now desire more detailed information and wish to participate and take responsibility for their own care.

In spite of this trend towards openness there is little information about what actually happens, and how many families with dying children do communicate freely. A recent study of children with cancer suggests it may still be relatively few, as only 19 per cent of this sample of families and children mutually acknowledged the approach of the child's death (Goldman and Christie 1993).

It seems that although many professionals now value open communication, it can be more difficult to achieve in practice than in theory. Even experienced staff who overtly expressed the wish to be open, have been observed to use distancing tactics regularly (Maguire 1985). Some reasons which have been identified for this include fear of being blamed, fear of handling the unknown, fear of unleashing a powerful re-action, and fear of expressing their own emotions (Buckman 1984).

COMMUNICATING WITH CHILDREN

I know I'm going to die. I know I'm going to heaven because I've been there already, Jesus showed me round. It was a lovely place. But I don't know how I'm going to get there. It's the moment of death that worries me.

The 13-year-old boy who said this had been ill for about ten years. Throughout his illness, his mother had always given him appropriate information about his treatment and the possible outcome of his disease. He was, therefore, ready to talk about the anxieties that were uppermost at each point, on what he saw as his long journey towards death. His example illustrates four key aspects to effective communica-ion with children about death:

(1) the need for an awareness of the developmental level of the child;

(2) the value of appreciating the existing communication system within the family;

(3) the realization that effective communication can reduce anxiety;

(4) the choice of the medium of communication most easily used by the child. In this illustration it was verbal.

It is easy to fall into the trap of thinking of communication as though it were one way, from adults to children, with factual content only. In fact, it is always two way, for even if an adult gives some information to a child there will be some feedback from the child's response. Sometimes the adult fails to recognize the child's response, especially if it is non-verbal; it is also possible for the adult to choose not to acknowledge it, perhaps because this would mean confronting difficult issues. What is more, there is a need for everyone to communicate feelings as well as facts. At one level, feelings can best be understood by non-verbal means; the hug that means more than a thousand words but some feelings can be expressed only in words. 'I'm not worried about myself when I die, it's my mum and dad I worry about.'

CHILDREN'S CONCEPTS

Concepts of illness

Children's ideas about illness are important. Eiser (1985) has discussed this and draws upon two distinct approaches. One is sociological and suggests that children learn sick role behaviour from others, especially their mothers. The other approach is cognitive, with proponents arguing that children's concepts follow the stages put forward by Piaget (Bibace and Walsh 1980) with an increasing move from concrete thinking towards the abstract. In a related study, Simmeonsson *et al.* (1979) found that sick children's concepts of illness went from the global, often reflecting magical thinking 'you get ill when you kiss old people', through to the more concrete idea that illness is related to specific actions, and finally to the more general in which principles were invoked. Brewster (1982) found that many children under the age of 7 years thought that they were ill because of something they had done. The complex nature of children's understanding in these areas is stressed in the recent literature (Bluebond-Langner 1994, Frangoulis *et al.* 1996).

Concepts of death

The concept of death is complex; children do not go to bed one night without a concept of death and wake up next morning with one. One reason for the gradual development of understanding of death is that the concept itself is built up of a number of components.

Kane (1979) identified nine components, listing them as follows, with the average ages at which they were attained in her sample:

(1)	realization	all 3-year-olds
(2)	separation	5 years
(3)	immobility	5 years
(4)	irrevocability	6 years
(5)	causality	6 years
(6)	dysfunctionality	6 years
(7)	universality	7 years
(8)	insensitivity	8 years
(9)	appearance	12 years

Other studies have attempted to establish the age at which some or all of these components emerge, both in healthy children (Lansdown and Benjamin 1985) and those with leukaemia (Clunies-Ross and Lansdown 1988). There were large individual differences in these studies and it is always as well to remind ourselves that it is dangerous to generalize too readily from research averages to any one child.

Matthew is a good example of a developing, but incomplete understanding. He was almost five when he said to his mother that he did not want to be an angel. He went on,

'Doctors can't make everyone better, can they?'
'No but they try very hard.'
'They can't make me better. But Jesus will make me better with love and kisses because Jesus doesn't give pricks. Then he'll send me back to you and daddy.'

We can make some guarded generalizations from the studies which are helpful in practice. Children almost always know more than most adults think they do. Separation is an aspect of death which is appreciated very early and is often a significant fear. We should be careful about accepting what a child says at face value, for there is often a degree of misunderstanding that can be masked by words.

Alongside the concept of death goes the concept of heaven. Many children have some notion of an afterlife, even if there has been no teaching of religion at home.

When Geraldine, a six-year-old whose parents were firm atheists who had forbidden any religious instruction, was told she was likely to die soon, she immediately assumed she would go to heaven and complained to her mother that she would be lonely there. 'Will you', she asked, 'be able to visit me in heaven like you visited me in hospital?'

There is an explanation for this in terms of developmental psychology. The idea that there is nothing after death is abstract and at this age children think in very concrete terms. It often seems to them that dying is a journey, and perhaps it is not surprising that they should see it this way, since so much of their lives so far has been predicated on journeys: from home to school, from home to hospital, from one hospital to another.

Concept of the stages of their illness

Along with considering the child's understanding of death and illness in general, we should also be aware of their ideas of themselves in relation to their own illness. These also develop with time and can be described in five stages, which can give some guidelines about the content of communication that can be expected.

1. *I am ill.* For some children, those with cancer for example, there is a more or less clear-cut beginning to the illness although there may be a grey period before the diagnosis. For others, with a progressive disease for example, the realization is likely to be more gradual but it is eventually reached.

2. *I have an illness that can kill people.* Some children reach this stage simply because they hear a word like leukaemia and

know perhaps rather vaguely that it is associated with death. Others are told by their parents, if for no other reason than to help explain why the treatment given is so awful. 'If you don't have this you'll die'.

But the understanding that comes at this stage is virtually academic and it is possible that some children do not believe what they are told. After all, Dad said last week that if I didn't tidy my bedroom he'd kill me but he didn't really mean it. It is only when Stage 3 is reached, that the full realization sinks in.

3. *I have an illness that can kill children.* When there are three boys with cystic fibrosis in a school one summer term and only two in the autumn, the remaining two have had the clearest possible lesson. We should always be on guard for the ripples that come to a ward or the special school class when a death occurs.

4. *I am never going to get better.* This may follow on quite quickly after Stage 3, or it may take some time. It is almost always associated with depression, a resignation to the continuance of the present state, whatever that may be. It does not, however, imply that children know that their death is imminent. That comes with Stage 5.

5. *I am going to die.* Some authors suggest that all children from about three upwards are capable of reaching this stage (Bluebond-Langner 1978). Within the normal canons of scientific enquiry the hypothesis is untestable but one must be open to the possibility that even very young children may have a full understanding not only of death, but of their own death.

At first, when children know they are ill, they need an explanation of the nature of the illness and the treatment. This must, of course, be tailored to the child's developmental level but the most common errors come in giving too little, rather than too much information.

Felicity was 12 when a life-threatening illness was diagnosed. She was living with her parents abroad, and the whole family suddenly moved to London so that she could have medical care. Her father insisted that she be told nothing more than that she had bad influenza. Felicity herself communicated her needs by screaming after a couple of days, 'You're lying . . . you must tell me the truth, you must'.

Learning about the severity of the illness will depend very largely on the nature of the condition, and generalizations are hard to make here. Children will often learn for themselves about Stage 3, that their illness can kill children and it is at this time that the focus should be more on what the child communicates to us, and responding to their needs, than on giving information. At this time and during Stages 4 and 5 comes the question of whether or not to tell children that they will die.

COMMUNICATION SYSTEMS WITHIN THE FAMILY

Just as one must acknowledge the child's developmental level, so we can only work within the families' own existing communication system and respect it; the arrogance of doing otherwise is likely to be counterproductive.

Working with an open system seems easy. If there is an expectation that people will be open in what they say, whatever the topic, then those matters concerning illness and death will form part of the same pattern. While this is so, even the most open families can find talking to a child about his own death very difficult. They also may require considerable awareness to pick up the cues that the children may give.

Christopher's parents held nothing back and their verbal and non-verbal communication with their six-year-old son was a model of how to do it. But towards the end, it was only through a careful observation of Christopher's drawings and the stories he told to accompany them, that they tuned in to his fears.

The notion of mutual pretence is often employed, when parents pretend they are not concerned because they do not want to worry their children, and children pretend they are not worried because they do not want to upset their parents.

A mature articulate ten-year-old girl, dying from a Wilms' tumour, indicated an awareness of her situation through her creation of an elaborate family tree, and concern with family photo albums, but she conformed to the family's protective pattern by not talking openly with anyone up to her death.

One way of tackling the problem presented by such a system is to go for it headlong: if one confronts the parents openly with the suggestion that they may be using this approach, they will often agree that they are. It is then possible, with parental permission, to take this up with the child and, thus, to allow parents and child to communicate with an adult while retaining the mutual pretence between each other. To critics who level accusations of collusion, one can respond that this compromise frees up both parents and children to communicate in ways that may be, for them, the best possible.

Another approach is to offer opportunities to children to communicate obliquely. Teachers and play specialists have a particular role to play here for the form of communication is often through play or school-work.

Robert was a bright 12-year-old with leukaemia who had been told by his parents that he was ill but that his illness was not serious. He had known several children on his ward die. He asked the ward teacher if he could do a project and the project he chose was 'blood'; a topic allowing him ample opportunity to ask all the questions he needed to.

The family who practise systems of denial and avoidance present the hardest problems of all, for they will not acknowledge even the notion of mutual pretence. For them, the least said by anyone, the better. While it is not difficult to understand the reason for this stance it can be stressful for professionals who can see the unmet needs on both sides. The oblique opportunities mentioned above may be a solution, but even they can be blocked by some parents. A direct confrontation may be of value but it is more likely than not to lead to further barriers being erected. One approach to effect change is to encourage parents to join a parents' group when it is possible that other parents put forward views which may be challenging but which will be perceived as more valid because they come from people with experience.

WAYS OF COMMUNICATING

One of the main aims of encouraging communication with children is to help them reduce their anxiety. It is hard for adults to appreciate not only how anxious children can be, but also what misapprehensions they may have which fuel worries.

One conversation overheard in a playroom illustrates this:

'What are you in for?'
'My eyes, I've got a squint.'
'Do you know how they mend eyes in this hospital?'
'No.'
'First they cut your head off, then they mend your eyes, then they sew your head back on again.'

Children with leukaemia, knowing their blood count is low, can be worried when they have a finger prick, for this is taking away precious blood which is, to them, already low. Children with a degenerative disease may invoke all manner of fantasies to explain their reduced performance. The more children can understand and anticipate what is going to happen to them, the less anxious they will be when it occurs.

One question frequently asked concerns timing: if I prepare my child for a nasty experience well in advance, this will only give more time for worrying. If I give the information just before, there will be no time to take it in and ask questions. A rule of thumb is that the older the child, the longer can be the time of preparation, although individual differences can be taken into account.

Play

Play is an excellent way both of preparing children, and of approaching feelings. Sometimes it is enough simply to observe free play, the children who constantly enact hospital scenes involving unpleasant procedures are not uncommon. Many children can play out fantasies, play at procedures (before and after), and play through anger. It is relatively easy to provide appropriate play material but harder for staff without training in psychotherapy to interpret play and it is better not to try, unless there is professional back-up.

Emily presented a serious preparation problem. She was two-and-a-half and had to have an arm amputated from the shoulder. The work with Emily was carried out by the play specialist who found a doll with a removable arm. Many games were played with this doll and then further games with an arm having been removed. Care was taken not to give the message that the arm could be replaced, and Emily's attention was drawn to the absence of an arm during the play. As far as could be told she coped well with her loss.

Surgery and procedures lend themselves well to the photo album with commentary approach. Dolls and teddy bears can also be used, although the latter provided an example of how literally some children think.

One ward team uses a teddy to explain the insertion of a central venous catheter, and for most children this has proved to be helpful, but at least one child was convinced that after she had the catheter, she too would be covered in short brown hairs, like the teddy.

Roger was just five-years-old and seemed intensely preoccupied with his illness. He refused to draw or to tell stories but said he would play Lego. We built a room which he announced was a laboratory. This led on to an imaginary conversation about people whose blood was being tested which led to a discussion of the implications of their illness if treatment were unsuccessful. He said, flatly, that they would die. Here at last was an opportunity to ask him outright if he thought he was going to die. He said sadly that he thought he would and added that he did not want to. Once that point had been reached we were able further to take up his anxieties.

Art

Drawing and painting, both easily accessible to most children, provide both opportunities and pitfalls. As in play, children can communicate specific messages.

Christopher, six-years-old when he died, drew a small boat tossed in a storm, supported by two large whales.

Stephens-Parker (unpublished data) asked children to draw themselves in hospital, and siblings were asked to draw their brother or sister. There was a striking difference between the two sets of pictures: siblings drew a child surrounded by staff and visitors; the sick children drew themselves in bed, isolated. She also compared the use of colour in pictures drawn by children with leukaemia, with those attending the dental department, and a healthy comparison group. There was a highly significant difference with the leukaemic children using far fewer colours. A discussion of a system of scoring family drawings is given in Spinetta and Deasy-Spinetta (1981). The pitfall with drawings is that it is easy to misinterpret and overinterpret them in an unscientific and dangerous way.

Talking

Oral communication can take many forms on a continuum from the direct to the oblique.

The most direct question the author has put to a patient was to ask when he thought he would die. The reply was 'in about a week' which turned out to be true and allowed a free discussion of the implications of death.

Another teenager, when asked if he was worrying about what was happening to him replied 'I know exactly what you are talking about but I don't want to discuss it, thank you.' He clearly did know, as his mother found his will in his diary after he died, but he made the choice not to talk at the time.

A more oblique example came from a girl in early December when she told her parents not to bother to buy her any Christmas presents.

WHEN DEATH APPROACHES

If death is not imminent, it can be better to act as if a cure is still hoped for, or in cases where the children know there is no cure, as if death is far in the future. To tell a child that he or she may die within the next four years may raise anxiety rather than allaying it.

However, when the time is nearer, the aim is to enable each child and family to face the inevitable, with as little anxiety and fear as possible, to be able to give and receive support, to express their needs and feelings, and to die, or for the family to live on, without regrets. Awareness of the child's level of understanding, the family's style of communication, and of different ways of approaching the topic should help the professional with this task.

Three-year-olds often benefit not from talk of death but from reassurance that there will always be someone to look after them. Slightly older children may take the imminent possibility of death surprisingly calmly but will need the opportunity to talk through the implications. As children approach their teens, there may be more fear and more anger. This does not mean that death should be denied, only that even more care be taken in offering further chances to talk.

If a child has been given full information about their treatment and the nature of their illness, then suddenly to stop telling the truth is likely to arouse considerable anxiety. This may be indicated by a change in mood. It often takes the form of becoming withdrawn and preoccupied, in extreme cases, stopping talking, eating, and playing. The child's fears and fantasies of the unknown are almost always worse than the reality, however bad that may seem to an adult. Talking with the children about death, and their worries, offers them the chance to express their feelings, relieves their sense of isolation, and gives them the opportunity of fulfilling any plans, and saying goodbye.

The long-term effect on parents of not telling the truth can also be considerable.

Max deteriorated suddenly at home and was rushed to hospital. As he was carried into the ambulance, he asked his father if he was dying. His father had not talked about the possibility of death before and, thrown by the question, answered that he was not. Max died in the ambulance and many months afterwards his father castigated himself because in his words 'My last words to my son were a lie.'

CONCLUSION

Claire Mulholland published a book of poems, written to her dead daughter, in 1974. The shortest was,

> Worst of all was the agony
> of not knowing
> what you knew.

If we can use every means at our disposal to communicate with children and to allow them to communicate with us, at least some of this fog-like agony will be dispelled.

REFERENCES

Bibace, R. and Walsh, M. (1980). Development of children's concepts of illness. *Paediatrics*, **66**, 912–17.

Bluebond-Langner, M. (1978). *The private worlds of dying children*. Princeton University Press, New Jersey.

Bluebond-Langner, M. (1994). A child's view of death. *Current Paediatrics*, **4**, 253–57.

Brewster, A. B. (1982). Chronically ill children's concepts of their illness. *Paediatrics*, **69**, 355–62.

Buckman, R. (1984). Breaking bad news: why is it still so difficult? *British Medical Journal*, **288**, 1597–9.

Chesler, M. A., Paris, J., and Barbarin, O. A. (1986). 'Telling' the child with cancer: parental choices to share information with ill children. *Journal of Pediatric Psychology*, **11**, 497–515.

Clunies-Ross, C. and Lansdown, R. (1988). Concepts of death, illness and isolation found in children with leukaemia. *Child: Care, Health and Development*, **14**, 373–86.

Eiser, C. (1985). *The psychology of childhood illness*. Springer-Verlag, New York.

Frangoulis, S., Jordan, N., and Lansdown, R. (1996). Children's concept of an afterlife. *British Journal of Religious Education*, **18**, 114–23.

Goldman, A. and Christie, D. (1993). Children with cancer talking about their own death, with their families. *Paediatric Haematology and Oncology*, **10**, 223–31.

Kane, B. (1979). Children's concepts of death. *Journal of Genetic Psychology*, **134**, 141–53.

Kendrick, C., Culling, J., Oakhill, T., and Mott, M. (1987). Children's understanding of their illness and its treatment within a paediatric oncology unit. *Association of Child Psychology and Psychiatry*, **8**, 2–5.

Lansdown, R. and Benjamin, G. (1985). The development of the concept of death in children aged 5–9 years. *Child: Care, Health and Development*, **11**, 13–20.

Maguire, P. (1985). Barriers to psychological care of the dying. *British Medical Journal*, **291**, 1711–13.

Mulholland, C. (1973). *I'll dance with the rainbows*. Partick Press, Glasgow.

Simeonsson, R., Buckley, L., and Monson, L. (1979). Conceptions of illness causality in hospitalized children. *Journal of Pediatric Psychology*, **4**, 77–84.

Spinetta, J. J. and Deasy-Spinetta, P. (ed.) (1981). *Living with childhood cancer*. C.V. Mosby, St Louis.

Spinetta, J. J., Swarner, J. A., and Sheposh, J. P. (1981). Effective parental coping following the death of a child from cancer. *Journal of Pediatric Psychology*, **6**, 251–63.

6

Provision of care

Ann Goldman and David Baum

Mortally ill children and their families need a flexible system of support from a broad spectrum of services to meet their needs: they need to be cared for day and night throughout the weeks, months, or years of illness; they need respite, palliative, and terminal care at home, in hospital, and elsewhere. The families' own resources, support from friends and the wider family, the diagnosis and length of illness, will all influence how much and what type of professional support is needed, and where it is most appropriately given.

Services for children who are dying must help the family cope with their child's physical deterioration and increasing dependence. They should include the relief of emotional, social, and spiritual distress as well as the physical and practical needs of the child and family, which may be constantly changing and in need of frequent reassessment. Time is precious and the quality of daily life paramount. While this type of care for children embodies the hospice philosophy, it is important to emphasize that, although it may be offered in a hospice, it can be delivered anywhere; in the home and during hospital admission, as well as in purpose-built facilities.

Life-threatening and life-limiting illness in childhood are rare. It is perhaps for this reason that the provision of care has not been planned systematically, but developed sporadically and fortuitously in response to individual initiatives.

Some recent initiatives have addressed the task of assessing the needs of children and families in detail, evaluating the different aspects of care being provided now and assessing the services which are needed for the future (While *et al.* 1996, ACT/RCPCH 1997, Thornes 1998). They suggest the provisions each child and family might expect (Table 6.1) and pathways forward, for those commissioning services for families and for professionals providing care are recommended.

However, since the services available in this country at the moment remain so variable, with no common framework,

Table 6.1   What every child and family should expect

1   To receive a flexible service according to a care plan, which is based on individual assessment of their needs, with reviews at appropriate intervals.

2   To have their own named keyworker to co-ordinate their care and provide access to appropriate professionals across the network.

3   To be included in the caseload of a paediatrician in their home area and have access to local clinicians, nurses and therapists skilled in children's palliative care and knowledgeable about services provided by agencies outside the NHS.

4   To be in the care of an identified lead consultant paediatrician expert in the child's condition.

5   To be supported in the day-by-day management of their child's physical and emotional symptoms and to have access to 24-hour care in the terminal stage.

6   To receive help in meeting the needs of parents and siblings, both during the child's illness and during death and bereavement.

7   To be offered regular respite which includes nursing care and symptom management, ranging from parts of a day to longer periods.

8   To be provided with medications, oxygen, specialized feeds and all disposable items such as feeding tubes, suction catheters and stoma products through a single source.

9   To be provided with housing adaptations and specialist equipment for use at home and school, in an efficient and timely manner without recourse to several agencies.

10 To be given assistance in procuring benefits, grants, and other financial help.

each family, their situation, and the facilities available for them, must be assessed individually. If the family have a key person who knows them and their network of carers well, he or she will be in an ideal position to assess the situation, and help introduce and co-ordinate appropriate facilities as they are needed. She or he will be able to spend time with the family considering the different options available, subsequently liaising between the professionals, smoothing communication, and clarifying individual roles and responsibilities.

As a child's illness progresses and the family and professionals become aware that they are entering the terminal stages, ideally the family should have a choice as to where the child should be cared for. While most families would, in principle, prefer this to be at home, they should also have access to a paediatric ward in hospital or a children's hospice. A genuine choice only exists if all these options are available and if the family are confident that they will have sufficient help available, at all times, for symptom management and psychosocial support wherever they are.

CARE AT HOME

During the child's illness, most families prefer to spend as much of their time as possible at home, in their neighbourhood. Although they may need respite care facilities during the course of the illness (see Chapter 7), many hope they will be able to be at home when the child dies. In this way, the child ends his or her life among the people he or she knows best, in familiar surroundings, while the family maintain control over at least their own domestic affairs. There is the possibility of brothers, sisters, neighbours, and members of the wider family remaining involved. Evidence suggests that the long-term problems of bereaved parents and siblings may be reduced when they have been involved in caring for the dying child at home (Lauer *et al.* 1989).

Considerable responsibilities fall on the parents whose child dies at home. They have to manage both the practical and emotional difficulties day in, day out, and strong professional support is vital. Such support may be provided through a combination of the primary health-care team, specialist nurses, and general community nursing services with back-up from the local or specialist hospital usually available (ACT/RCPCH 1997).

Most family doctors have had little experience caring for dying children and, unlike staff with a special interest in palliative care, this may be an area in which they feel relatively unskilled. The doctor may know the family well and have been involved throughout the child's illness; on the other hand, he or she may have had little recent contact, particularly if much of the child's treatment has been in hospital. The primary health-care team may feel that the hospital staff, recognizing the fatal nature of the child's disease, have abandoned the family and referred them back to the community at a late stage, imposing the burden of care upon them unreasonably. Some family doctors readily accept the challenge to acquire new skills and the emotional input required; others are uncomfortable with the unusual situation, the distress, and the commitment of time required. It is important, therefore, for those who rarely encounter children who are dying, to have ready access to specialist experience and skills required. Such back-up and resources have not been available in the past, and although the situation is improving, it can still be a problem.

Domiciliary nurses offer an important part of the spectrum of hospice care for children. In 1996, a total of 495 community paediatric nurses were identified, making up about 60 specialist and about 100 general teams. The majority of the general teams are funded by the NHS, but the funding of the specialist teams comes mostly from charitable sources. These specialist nursing teams include paediatric oncology specialist nurses, cystic fibrosis specialist nurses and other individual nurses who look after children with metabolic disorders and some conditions leading to major organ failure, such as heart, liver, and renal disease.

The general teams comprise community paediatric nurses who may not have had special training in paediatric palliative nursing, but may take on the care of such children in their area if they arise. There are teams of community paediatric nurses employed by a total of 19 NHS Trusts in

England. However this still means there are around 200 trusts providing community services but no paediatric team (Health Committee Report 1997).

There are a number of other related posts. The Sargent Cancer Care provides 45 social workers throughout the UK for children with cancer. The Muscular Dystrophy Group funds 14 family care officers based at centres providing a service for neuromuscular diseases. At present there is only one paediatrician with a specialist interest in palliative care, and this post is also funded by charity.

Staff working in the community, particularly those with a disease-specific remit, prove to be of enormous value to the families. They serve as a key person for the family, and work closely with the primary health care teams and hospital centres. The majority of families caring for children with cancer now have this type of sophisticated support system. However, it is not available for everyone, especially those families caring for children with unusual degenerative disorders. It is these families, rare in their locality, but numerically substantial nationally, who look to their primary health care teams, to the voluntary agencies, and to the children's hospice facilities for care and support, and for whom a more co-ordinated approach is needed in the future (ACT/RCPCII 1997).

CHILDREN'S HOSPICES

Since the first children's hospice, Helen House, opened in Oxford in 1982, twelve others have been established (Listed in Appendix E). The majority take children from their immediate locality but some accept children from anywhere in the country. There are also a number of other children's hospice initiatives at variable stages of development (details available from ACT).

The children's hospices each have a multidisciplinary staff team and offer respite, palliative care, and bereavement support. Some are able to offer, additionally, a degree of domiciliary nursing support when a child is dying at home. The buildings vary in detail but all aim to provide a warm and supportive atmosphere in an informal, non-institutional setting. They have individual rooms for the sick children, offering care for 7–12 children at a time. There are rooms for families to stay, hydrotherapy, room and equipment for play, and space for peace.

Whilst adult hospices care mainly for people with malignant diseases, the children's hospices have provided care for children with a much wider range of conditions. The majority of work constitutes respite care for families with children with progressive neurological disease and other life-threatening genetic disorders. A smaller number of children with malignant disease have used this service: this includes, particularly, children with brain tumours in whom a more chronic and disabling phase is likely. The range of disorders of the children staying at Helen House reflects this pattern (see Table 6.2).

Table 6.2 Diagnostic categories of 147 children admitted to Helen House between November 1982 and December 1986

	Number	Per cent of total
CNS degenerative disorders	56	38
Malignant disease	30	20
Mucopolysaccharidoses	25	17
Neuromuscular disorders	16	11
Congenital abnormalities	14	10
Others	6	4

Data from Dominica (1987).

The established children's hospices are busy and continue to experience increasing referrals. In some cases, the children's hospices, in effect, take on the role of key worker for the families in their care. The families gain not only from care during their stay, but also have their sense of isolation relieved even when they return home. However, children's hospice facilities are very costly to build, equip, and run. Virtually all this money has, up till now, been raised from voluntary contributions.

HOSPITAL CARE

Some families choose not to care for their child at home but prefer, as death approaches, to return to the hospital. Often they will have had close ties with the ward over many years, know the staff well, and feel comfortable and confident there. For some children whose care in hospital has been directed towards cure, it is only at a very late stage that it becomes apparent that death is inevitable, and at this stage it may be felt that transfer would be inappropriate. The Department of Health document *Welfare of children and young people in hospital* specifically offers guidance for good practice in caring for children dying in hospital.

It can be difficult for staff who are usually geared to aggressive medical care to adjust to the different priorities and pace required in caring for a child who is dying. Stopping unnecessary observations, ensuring privacy, and offering support whilst not intruding are important skills. Families should feel that staff are comfortable just being alongside them, without needing to do anything, but not that the attentions offered to a child who may be cured are being withdrawn.

Some aspects of care can become complicated by hospital bureaucracy, and policy needs to be thought out ahead of time and made clear to all staff. Some hospitals facilitate this through a multidisciplinary Terminal Care Committee. Areas to consider are including parents in the care of their child's body, respecting the traditions of different cultures, allowing families adequate time with their dead child, providing a place of privacy to grieve, and ready access to mortuary viewing areas.

SUMMARY

It is clear that the services available at the moment are inadequate and unevenly distributed. They are unable to meet the suggestions of the ACT/RCPCH report and Department of Health documents, for the families whose children are mortally ill. All the children's hospices and many of the professionals working in the community are funded by charities. It is to be hoped that priority will be given to developing the services and identifying the funding to fill the large gaps which still exist in the provisions for palliative care for children.

REFERENCES

ACT (Association for children with life-threatening or terminal conditions and their families) and RCPCH (Royal College of Paediatrics and Child Health) (1997). *A guide to the development of Children's Palliative Care Services.*

Dominica, F. (1987). The role of the hospice for the dying child. *British Journal of Hospital Medicine*, October, 334–42.

Health Committee Report (1997). Health Services for children and young people in the community: Home and School, Available from PO Box 276, London SW8 5DT, 0171 873 9090.

Lauer, M. E., Mulhern, R. K., Schell, M. J., and Camitta, B. M. (1989). Long-term follow-up of parental adjustment following a child's death at home or hospital. *Cancer*, **63**, 988–94.

Thornes, R. (1998) on behalf of Department of Health. Evaluation of the Pilot Project programme for children with life threatening illnesses. Available from NHS response line 0541 555 455 or DOH Stores, PO Box 410, Wetherby LS23 7LN.

While, A., Citrone, C., and Cornish, J. (1996). *Executive summary of a study of the needs and provisions for families caring for children with life limiting incurable disorders*. Department of Health, London.

7

Practical issues

Jean Simons

The awareness of death in the shorter or longer term is very real for the families of children with life-threatening or life-limiting disorders, and the need for adjustment, planning, and support is vital. Types of help required and their sources will vary. They will depend upon whether plans have to be made at the outset of the child's life, when the condition becomes apparent, or whether the situation is of a healthy child becoming acutely or chronically, and then terminally ill. Also, of course, the age of the child during illness and terminal events will have a great influence upon the family. If the whole event from diagnosis to death is played out during young babyhood, the child's and family's needs will be different from those of a family where the child's deterioration occurs gradually and the child may reach teenage or young adulthood before death.

This chapter will outline some of the key financial and practical problems arising during the child's illness. The second section will focus on the practical issues which face all families at the time of their child's death.

THE CHILDREN ACT AND LOCAL AUTHORITIES

The Children Act (1989), in operation since 14th October 1991, lays a duty on local authorities to provide support for 'children in need', including 'such provision as they consider appropriate'. The theme of the Act is that parents and local authorities should work in partnership as far as possible, and the philosophy of the Act is for support to parents in caring for their child, with 'stronger rights for parents and children and less interference by the State in the lives of families'.

A child is defined by the Children Act (1989) as being in need if:

(a) he is unlikely to achieve or maintain or to have the opportunity of achieving or maintaining a reasonable standard of health or development, without the provisions for him of services by a local authority under this Part (of the Act);

(b) his health or development is likely to be significantly impaired, or further impaired, without the provision for him of such services; or

(c) he is disabled.

Many professionals working within the Children Act continue to be concerned that under-resourced authorities will not be able to meet their obligations towards all children in need. Before the present Act, there was a duty upon local authorities to assess numbers and requirements of disabled children in their area (Chronically Sick and Disabled Persons Act 1970), but provision was not mandatory and varied widely. Some boroughs and authorities had appropriate services but others, which perceived themselves to be in great financial difficulties had very inadequate provisions.

ORGANIZING AND OBTAINING HELP

To obtain benefits, practical help, and respite care, families often have to be quite demanding to discover and receive the help which is available to them, and some families do not ever get it. Several researchers from voluntary groups (Hearn and Evans 1990; Lavery 1988; Thornes 1987) share the conclusions that appropriate, effective, flexible help from professionals is often difficult to co-ordinate or even obtain.

In Christine Lavery's survey only 23 per cent of families questioned were receiving any practical care at home. Problems identified by families in one study were, as may be expected, concern over the child's symptoms, the course of the illness, the child's ultimate death, where it would be, how it would be, and how the family would manage. Some families talked of the impact of the illness on the lives of the well siblings. The study identified the main parental worry as anxiety about their capacity to continue coping with the child's illness if their own health failed. The financial burden on families was great, often because bread-winners had become unemployed, had chosen or been forced to give up work, or had to cut back drastically on the hours worked. Over time, the cost of such things as nappies, travelling, heating, laundry, household alterations, and special equipment could become very expensive for any particular family, especially if more than one child were affected.

Typically, many families experienced difficulty in identifying and obtaining appropriate help, and this added to their distress. Half of the families had contact with a 'knowledgeable professional' who had helped them to mobilize available sources of help. Others had gleaned information in a piecemeal way from voluntary societies or well-informed friends. This highlights the need for centralized, co-ordinated, easily available information. The researchers who conducted the study, developed the concept of 'cornerstone care' for families of children with life-threatening and terminal illness, very similar to Thorne's (1987) concept of the 'key worker'. The cornerstone carer was the person the parents identified as the professional most closely involved with them, who had been able to help them co-ordinate services, and to give support and care over time, whilst still enabling them to feel in control of their own lives.

The Joint Working Party Guide to the Development of Children's Palliative Care Services (1997) validates and re-emphasizes the need for co-ordination, communication and flexibility between health, social services, and education departments in planning, commissioning, and provision of services.

FINANCIAL BENEFITS—A MINEFIELD

There are some benefits relevant to most families caring for a child or young adult with a life-threatening or life-limiting illness which are discussed briefly here. (More detail is provided in Appendix D.) The only benefit not means-tested or taxable is the Disability Living Allowance (DLA); all others are financially means-tested. The DLA is the tax-free benefit introduced in April 1992. For families on Income Support extra premiums may be available, relevant to individual circumstances.

Families may be well advised to contact a Welfare Rights Officer at their local Social Services Department, or a knowledgeable volunteer at their local Citizens' Advice Bureau to help them work out which benefits they are eligible for. Two leaflets which are easily available and set out clearly and helpfully the chief benefits which families may like to consider are:

(1) the Contact-A-Family leaflet entitled *Child disability benefits and other sources of help*;

(2) the Research Trust for Metabolic Diseases in Children (August 1991) *Family information leaflet*.

The need for some families eventually to appeal for the provision of this and other benefits, carries the suggestion of begging for help, an unacceptable stigma to many families.

Professionals working with families claiming benefits need to be prepared to take on the advocacy role to help families who may already feel exhausted, isolated, and stigmatized to gain what (fairly meagre) provision may be helpful to them.

Additional help

Financial help may also be available from other sources, or as benefit in kind from some organizations. The Family Fund, the Family Welfare Association, Local Health Authorities, and Social Services Departments may help with nursing aids, adaptations, appliances, nappies, or wheelchairs. Provision varies between boroughs and authorities. Loans from the Red Cross may be available and families should approach or be helped to approach their local authority for nursing aids, and their local occupational therapist, either via the Social Services Department or the local hospital, for such things as aids to daily living. Specific benefits to aid mobility may also be available, such as fares to hospital, orange badge schemes, and community transport schemes; Motability and RADAR (Royal Association for Disability and Rehabilitation) provide information about discounts and concessions on cars for disabled people.

Charities

Families may find themselves reliant on the provision available from various charities. There are many specialized organizations, all aiming to help families whose child suffers from the condition particular to their own interest. A very good source of information here is the organization Contact-A-Family. The Family Fund may be able to provide goods and services such as washing-machines, tumble-driers, or other equipment, and may also help towards the cost of a holiday for families who have a child whose life is threatened, but who are not eligible for help from any other specific charity.

RESPITE CARE

For families who take care of a seriously ill child at home, the opportunity for respite care is vital. However willingly and lovingly they assume the role of carers, it is essential to offer them some time away from the physically and emotionally exhausting tasks of care. For respite care to work, it has to have the confidence of both parents and children. Often lack of confidence in the skills or qualifications of the staff prevents parents taking up the option of care which would have benefited themselves and their family.

Lavery (1988) spoke of 'territorial injustice' in the provisions offered. Some families have suffered lack of immediate advice about the possibilities of respite care. Others

stated that they did not use respite care facilities locally
because these were totally inappropriate to their child's
needs, for example care on a geriatric ward or in a mental
health setting. Some local authorities and local groups offer
their own version of respite care through such services as
specialist baby-sitting, crossroads projects, etc. On the whole
these are not centrally co-ordinated and are necessarily
somewhat piecemeal according to local funding and enthu-
siasm. The survey highlighted the inflexibility and in-
adequacy of many statutory respite care facilities.

The respite care which parents valued most was the children's hospice provision. However, although there are now
eleven established hospices and several other local initiatives
for the future, these do not fulfil the needs for all the children
with life-threatening illnesses. Lavery (1988) comments
that the Griffiths Report (which calls for more parental
involvement and decision-making in community care) and the
Community Care Act may be a step in the right direction,
but both initiatives will founder unless the will is found
to fund generously and properly the model of respite care
which most parents value.

HOLIDAYS

Holiday homes and breaks are provided by charities, and can
be organized by the hospital or local authority social worker.
They are often in dedicated holiday homes in the UK or
abroad, which are specially equipped and available all year
round to families with a child suffering from a life-
threatening illness.

These homes provide a much needed and welcome break
for the whole family to be together. Unlike the hospices, they
do not offer medical or nursing care, although this is quickly
available if needed for the child. Care is usually provided by
the family themselves, but the opportunity for the family to
be away from their, perhaps, very stressful home environment, and be cared for themselves by the house staff, while
cooking and housework is done for them and baby-sitters are
available, can be a tremendous benefit.

ETHNIC-SENSITIVE PROVISION

Dugmore (1990) addresses the issue of incorrect assumptions made by medical and paramedical staff about the amount of understanding a parent may have if their first language is not English. Difficulties with medical jargon and some words which do not translate into languages other than English may lead to misunderstanding. Particular problems are, inappropriate use of family members as interpreters, and professionals' lack of knowledge of cultural issues, which may lead to misunderstanding, or ignoring of advice given if it appears unacceptable to a particular family's culture. Dugmore also highlights the paucity of written information available in languages other than English about some diseases.

Genetic counselling is a sensitive issue for many families, and particularly so in some cultures, which encourage marriage between blood relations, thus enhancing the chance of genetically-linked conditions. Many cultures which operate on an extended family system may prefer to derive most of their help and support from within their own family, which is entirely laudable if they are receiving the amount of help and advice which they need, in order to care appropriately for their child. It is important to be sure that benefits, provision of services, and respite care are equally accessible to any family whose first language is not English.

EDUCATION

One of the great normalizing factors in the life of all children, especially those who have a condition which is life-threatening, is the provision of schooling according to the child's age and ability. Jeffery (1990) states that many people do not value the point of education, seeing the concentration on schooling, homework, and academic effort as being potentially unkind to a child who may not have long to live and for whom effort may be difficult or painful. However, he argues that the whole point of treatment and efforts to normalize life, should not be to postpone dying but to prolong living and 'if all is tolerated, it may seem to the child that all is lost'. Education represents normality and normal expectations are reassuring to children who have a life-threatening illness. Teachers offer a respite from the sense of being different or unusual. It is normal to sit in a classroom with school-friends and to work towards shared goals. If a child is unable to attend school in the classroom with his or her school-friends, home tuition should be provided so that the child continues the contact with school-work. Individual schools and teachers may make efforts to arrange visits to the sick child in hospital or at home by school-friends and staff members but there is no statutory provision for this.

Unfortunately, there is a wide variation between local education authorities and many lack resources for home tutors. As long ago as 1978, the Warnock Report commenting on Hospital and Home Teaching Services, made a plea for unity of provision, but up to the present, local authorities have only power but not duty to provide education. Pleading financial pressure, many do not see the provision of such services as a priority. Future funding of educational services gives further cause for concern. The Education Reform Act (1988) devolves much expense to schools themselves, and out-of-school provision will become discretionary. Local management of schools makes them into rivals for 'customers' and special-needs children may fall between competing resources.

Professionals helping families through the maze of benefits and provision which may be available for their child have a duty to support the family in their determination to find appropriate education for their child. The Education Act (1981) provides for children to be assessed for special needs if it seems that their education will be adversely affected by an illness or disability. Once the needs have been assessed, a local or education authority 'must make appropriate arrangements to meet them and keep them under review'. An education authority may need to issue a formal statement of special educational needs which should guarantee the necessary provision. The 1993 Education Act (implemented

September 1994) sets out responsibilities of governing bodies of all schools in relation to children with special needs. A Code of Practice has been written for guidance to local authorities, explaining these responsibilities.

Day-care for under fives

Local authorities are required to provide day-care for children in need who are aged five or under. Day-care is defined as 'any form of care or supervised activity for children during the day'. It may, however, be hard for many local authorities who see themselves as financially hard-pressed to provide nursery or play-scheme placements for children whose needs are because of an illness or disability. Other specialist provision by local education authorities or local authorities such as peripatetic specialist teachers, Portage schemes, etc., may be affected by local budgets, local hospital trust status, or local purchaser/provider agreements. Professionals should be prepared to take an advocacy role with local authorities and local education authorities in these matters and a working knowledge of the relevant sections of the Children Act will be important.

PRACTICAL ISSUES AT THE TIME OF DEATH

Death in hospital

Families need, as far as possible, to be freed from fear of what is happening by being given frequent and exact information about what can be done, how and when, for their child. Parents often need help and encouragement to remain in control, to hold, talk to, or care for the child as much as they can, despite the possibly intimidating nature of the surroundings. After the child's death, the family should be able to spend as much time as they need with the child, taking part in such procedures as washing or dressing the child and should be encouraged freely to visit the child in the days following death. Care must be taken to observe the wishes of families of different ethnic and religious backgrounds as practices following a death may vary greatly, and if not sensitively observed, may cause the family added distress (see Chapter 8).

As long as no coroner's post-mortem is required, the family may, once the death has been registered, take the child's body home themselves. Usually the funeral director does this but families and staff may be unaware that the family may take the child themselves if they wish. The child can be taken in their own car and a coffin may be used, but is not essential.

Before a family leave the hospital following the death of their child, the consultant should make a firm appointment for a convenient time in the future, probably in about four to six weeks, to see the family again in the hospital if they so wish, particularly if a post-mortem has been performed, in order to explain and discuss the results.

Mementoes

It is important for staff members to recognize the importance of photographs of the child, particularly if the death is sudden or unexpected, and to ensure that these are taken if the family do not feel able to handle this themselves. Hand- and footprints of small children and locks of hair can also be taken. Some families may not wish to acknowledge the importance of such mementoes at this time, and it may be that staff should keep them discreetly in the child's file at the hospital, while assuring the parents that they will be available in future in they wish.

Post-mortems

If the child has been suffering from a chronic life-threatening disease it is unlikely that a post-mortem will be required for legal reasons, although occasionally this may happen. In this situation, the family have no choice and should receive as full an explanation as possible about the reasons and the inevitable short delay in making arrangements.

A more frequent possibility is that hospital staff may request a post-mortem to find out more details about the reason for the child's death and, particularly in the case of rare diseases to try to further medical knowledge. Requests and explanation should come from a senior doctor and be offered in such a way that parents do not feel under pressure to agree. Parents can refuse to agree to a post-mortem unless it is required by the coroner, in which case they have no choice.

Organ donation

If the child's death is imminent in hospital and if it has been sudden, perhaps as the result of an accident, permission may be sought to use a child's organs after death. This is a request which families sometimes anticipate; they may derive some satisfaction from feeling that through their child, they can help others. This is a subject which parents should be able to discuss thoroughly with relevant hospital staff before the child's death. Even if the child is dying from an illness which precludes using many of their organs it may be possible to transplant their corneas, and parents may wish to consider this option, or indeed the child or young person themselves may wish to consider this if they are aware of, and given the chance to discuss their own impending death.

Death at home

If the child is to die at home, it is likely that this is following a long illness. It is a shocking and disabling feeling for most parents to be, in effect, planning their child's death. Most parents needs a great deal of information and support if they are to feel confident that they can make their child's remaining life as comfortable and normal as possible. Almost all parents fear that they may be unable to cope with whatever symptoms the child may have and they need to know in specific detail what these are likely to be. They want to be able to express their fears and concerns and are often apologetic and guilty about mentioning such matters.

Parents need very clear information about what help they will be able to receive in caring for their child in terms of symptom-relief, nursing care, visits from their doctor, etc.

They need to be confident that they can get hold of someone they know and trust at any time of the day or night. It is good if professionals who are in a position to help parents can recommend before a child dies, that such things as photos, tape recordings, and videos provide extremely precious memories, and encourage families to think about these options. It is often very hard for parents as part of the process of acknowledging that the child's death is imminent to do these things, but later on they can be very important, both for themselves, siblings, and any future children.

Many parents feel that they have to act in certain ways very quickly after the death, and they need reassurance that there is nothing that has to be done in a hurry. If what they need most is time to be with their child, there is no need for any hasty action which they may regret later. It is helpful if parents can be encouraged to think how they might wish to handle things, for example being with the child, keeping him or her at home, including other family members and siblings, and dressing the child. They need to be as firm as they can in their wishes and not allow themselves to be railroaded by friends or relatives, however well-meaning, who may wish to assume the burden of arranging a funeral. Many families are unaware that if the child has died at home, it may be possible to keep the child at home, or to bring his or her body home again from the Chapel of Rest, prior to the funeral.

Registering the death

After a child's death, whether at home or in hospital, once parents have had as much time and privacy as they feel they need with their child, certain practical steps do have to be taken. If a child dies in hospital, the hospital doctor will sign the death certificate. If the child has died at home, the family doctor will usually do this. It is essential that the family and doctor have made clear arrangements for this ahead of time so that distress is avoided. Difficulties can occur if a locum is covering for the weekend and refuses to sign the certificate or a relative inadvertently dials 999 and ambulance staff begin resuscitation or take the child to a local accident and emergency department rather than the familar hospital.

Once the death certificate is signed, the child's death must be registered at the local registry office within 5 days. It is usual for a parent to register a child's death, but not essential. A relative, friend, or member of staff can do this, as long as they have the death certificate and appropriate information with them.

The following must be provided at the time of registration.

1. Certificate of the cause of death.
2. Date and place of death.
3. The child's full name, home address, date, and place of birth.
4. The parents' full names, home address, and occupations.
5. The Child Benefit Book and child's medical card if available, if not, they can be posted on later.

The registrar provides a certificate (sometimes called the green form) which is required by the funeral director before funeral arrangements can be made. Extra death certificates can be provided for a small fee. Once the certificate is issued, the family may make their own arrangements with a funeral director, regarding what happens to their child's body in the time leading up to the funeral.

FUNERALS

Although parents may find it very hard to talk about a funeral before the child has died, most will admit that they have had thoughts or fantasies about this. It is important for any professional helper to acknowledge with the family that this is normal, there is no need to feel guilt, and that it can be helpful for the family to think about and discuss. There is an increasing recognition now of the important rite of passage represented by a funeral. Parents of a pre-term or stillborn infant can now expect discussion of a thoughtful and appropriate service for their child, something which would not have been the case only a few years ago.

Parents need help to talk through their own beliefs, fears, wishes, and anxieties about burial and cremation, to help

them make an informed choice. They need to be encouraged
to talk to a number of funeral directors, not just to obtain
financial estimates but to try and decide who may be most
sympathetic to their needs. Families may already know of a
vicar or religious leader whom they would wish to conduct
a service, or they may not profess or practise a particular
religion themselves, and may need to know that it is quite
possible to organize a secular form of service and to involve
friends, family, and lay people in this (Spottiswoode 1991;
Albery 1992).

If the dying child has been part of a family where communication has been quite open, they may have expressed
their own wishes concerning the funeral such as whether
they favour burial or cremation, what they wish to wear, or
how they feel the ceremony should be conducted. If no
opinion or guidance is possible from the child, parents need
to think about and discuss the type of funeral which would
be appropriate for them. Although undoubtedly an occasion
for great sadness, many families wish to regard the funeral
service as a celebration of the child's life and accordingly may
be able to arrange a less solemn atmosphere through choos-
ing to wear bright clothes, choice of music and readings,
inclusion of the child's friends in the ceremony, perhaps
through the school choir or a particular music group (Walter
1990; Wilkinson 1991).

It is helpful to discuss with parents how they plan to
handle the matter of young children in the family attending
the funeral. Traditional, and no doubt well-meaning, advice
has been that a funeral is an upsetting experience for
young children. Research experience and anecdotal evidence
from families now leads most professionals to believe that,
upsetting though a funeral may be for all members of the
family, it is usually better for younger children to share what
is happening, than to feel further bewildered and shut-out
by not being involved. If children are old enough to be given
a choice and they do not wish to attend, then this should, of
course, be respected, but hopefully communication in the
family is such that the choice can be made after informed
discussion, and not in an atmosphere of exclusion.

Occasionally, a parent or family feel unable to arrange the child's funeral and wish to leave this to hospital staff, friends, or other members of the wider family. This should be discouraged as far as possible because parents almost invariably regret not having been in charge of the funeral arrangements themselves. If parents are unable to manage the practicalities of registration, there may be a person in the wider family or a member of the hospital staff who can do this for them, or support them whilst they carry out these tasks, but it is usually better if parents can themselves arrange the funeral.

Some families, in addition to a religious or secular ceremony, will wish to hold a wake or a party. Nearly all families will want to consider and discuss the provision of a suitable memorial for the child, which may be a physical object such as a headstone, a tree, or perhaps a piece of equipment at the child's school. Some families designate for themselves a place which was special to them, or the child; part of the garden, or perhaps a favourite picnic or play area.

AFTER THE FUNERAL

The help and support which the family may have valued before the child's death will still be needed after the funeral. A family who has coped for months or years with the exhausting task of caring for a sick child may be suddenly utterly bereft of their entire lifestyle and focus. Families may need reminding about and help with such miserable tasks as returning the Child Benefit Book, cancelling insurance policies, handing back any nursing equipment, aids, or adaptations, and cancelling any benefits which were coming into the home on behalf of the sick child.

Families may need reassurance that they will not lose all the help and support that they have received during their child's lifetime. It may be helpful for them to have written information about befriending, counselling, or support groups which they may not wish to take advantage of immediately, but which may be of interest or reassurance to them in the future. Most importantly families need a promise of future contact, even if it is anticipated that it will be infrequent or decreasing. It is not enough for a helper to offer availability to the family at their own initiative, as few have the energy or confidence to take that initiative. It is much better, indeed necessary, for a firm appointment to be made for an appropriate date in the future when an agreed form of contact, a visit, or a phone call will take place. At that contact it may be apparent that the family need some continuing help in their bereavement, and this can then be acknowledged and arranged, or, it may be that the family are coping well and that contact will provide the appropriate occasion to 'say goodbye'.

CONCLUSION

The involved professional can be of most help to a family if, as well as emphasizing, rightly, the symptom-relief and emotional support offered, he or she can also act as an informed advocate in the matter of practical issues.

Appropriate provision and consistent support are vital to a family caring for a child or young adult with a life-threatening illness. Financial benefits are not, on the whole, generous, respite care is of variable quality and availability, and entitlement to practical provision does not always seem consistent. Nevertheless, some extra, regular income in the form of a benefit, provision of labour-saving household goods or equipment, access to a much needed holiday, and confidence in what needs to be done at the time of death may make the difference between a family feeling burdened and despairing, or coping, as confidently as is possible, with their dying child.

REFERENCES

ACT "Children's Hospices: A Place for Living". Information Pack available from ACT, 65 St Michael's Hill, Bristol BS2 8BJ.
Albery, N. (1992). *The natural death handbook*, available through Natural Death Centre, 20 Heber Road, London NW2 6AA.

Contact-A-Family (1990). *Child disability benefits and other sources of help*, available from Contact-A-Family, 16 Strutton Ground, London SW1P 2HP.

Department for Education (1994). Special Educational Needs. A Guide for Parents.

Domenica, F. (1997). *Just my reflection.* Dartman, Longman and Todd, London.

Dugmore, J. (1991). Language lessons. *Community Care*, February, 24–6.

Dyer, C. (1991). *The Guardian*, 2nd October.

Hearn, J. and Evans, M. (1990). The Work of ACT; presented at the First National Conference on the Care of Children with Life Threatening Conditions, London.

HMSO (1970). *Chronically Sick and Disabled Person's Act.*

HMSO (1978). *Report of the Committee of Enquiry into the education of handicapped children and young people.* (Warnock Report.)

HMSO (1988). *Community care—an agenda for action.* (Griffiths Report.)

HMSO (1990). *National Health Service and Community Care Act.*

HMSO (1991). *The Children Act 1989—guidance and regulations.* In *Children with disabilities*, Vol. 6.

Joint Working Party (Association for children with life-threatening and terminal conditions and their families and Royal College of Paediatrics and Child Health) (1997). *A guide to the development of Children's Palliative Care Services.*

Jeffrey, P. (1990). In *Listen my child has a lot of living to do*, (ed. J. D. Baum, F. Dominica, and R. Woodward), pp. 133–7. Oxford University Press.

Lavery, C. (1988). *An investigation into respite care, needs and facilities offered to families of children suffering from mucopolysaccharide diseases.* Available from the Society for MPS Diseases, Motability, Gate House, Westgate, Harlow, Essex, CM10 20HR.

Research Trust for Metabolic Diseases in Children, (RTMDC) (1991). *Family information leaflet*, available from 53 Beam Street, Nantwich, Cheshire, CW5 5NF.

Spottiswoode, J. (1991). *Undertaken with love.* Robert Hale, London.

Thornes, R. (1987). *Care of dying children and their families*, available from National Association of Health Authorities (NAHA) Birmingham.

Walter, T. (1990). *Funerals and how to improve them.* Hodder and Stoughton, Sevenoaks.

Wilkinson, T. (1991). *The death of a child: a book for families.* Julia Macrae Books, London.

8

Spiritual and cultural aspects

Derek Bacon

A SHARED WORLD OF MEANING

'Let each child draw round his own hand, then write inside the outline the three things he likes best about himself, then talk to a friend about why these things matter, why her three things matter, and the different shapes of their hands.' (Clark 1991.)

These children are engaged in making sense of who they are and of how they relate to each other. They are building and sharing a world of meaning and identity. They are exploring their self-awareness and responding to the uniqueness of the other. The exercise gives us a glimpse of a lifelong quest which I would describe as the spiritual dimension of human existence.

The quest is individual and unique for each child. Different concerns will be carried according to temperament, the company of peers, and the society of significant adults. What each child makes of things will depend greatly upon how matters are ordered, the way of life in which he or she is nurtured. This way of life I would describe as the cultural dimension.

From such a simple sketching of terms, it should be clear how the spiritual and the cultural are interwoven, the one depending on the other, rather like adult and child.

While it is true that children, in their vulnerability, depend upon adults, we often forget that the reverse is equally, if differently, the case. All of us depend upon children to help us keep important things alive in our inner world, for the hint of what might be, for our feeling of belonging in and our sense of the rightness of the universe. Children are insistently alive, both energizing and exhausting their parents who depend upon them, perhaps only half knowingly, to carry much of the fantasy in the relationship that gave them birth, to fill the gap in what Winnicott (1965) has called their 'imaginative needs'. So when the life of a child of whatever age is threatened and the veil of taken-for-granted reality is torn away, the gap in those needs is exposed and a whole world of meaning stands in balance.

It is a world not only of the present, but one which reaches into the past memory, and future hope of the parent. It envelops the child and the family circle, and overlaps that of the health worker as well, giving the delivery of terminal care a potentially sharper edge. The sick child touches the child in us, and our world of meaning comes under threat of futility and emptiness when confronted with the child who is going to die. Detached and measured on the surface, we crumble a little underneath. For part of what makes us human at all is the need to make some sense of life by placing ourselves on a spiritual and cultural map. A great deal of what we allow ourselves to hope for is moulded by where we perceive ourselves to be on such a map.

MATTHEW

Matthew was in his early teens when he needed a heart–lung transplant. During what turned out to be his final admission to hospital, his mother and father kept themselves distanced from staff, while rarely actually leaving their son's side. Their distress was heightened when he let it be known that he felt he was going to die, and that there were matters he could not discuss with them but which he wanted someone to hear. Since the word 'god' had been mentioned, and since those who were most closely involved did not feel comfortable about such a conversation, it was suggested that he might be able to use the presence of a chaplain.

Matthew and his parents agreed, though at first he allowed them to speak on his behalf. Soon, however, he asked them to leave and over the next few encounters he revealed a rich and imaginative inner life. Some deeply hidden longings and fears found expression and, when acknowledged, saw resolution born of his own courage and maturity. A kind of tranquillity emerged which communicated to the parents. They began to see a son whom they had not known. They became less concerned about what he could want to say to a stranger and not to them, more aware of his need to articulate what was authentically his. Their grip on him was loosened. They grew in their openness to staff, and a change was observable in their treatment of one another. Ultimately, it was decided that Matthew could not be put on the active list for transplant. No such end is good, but, when death came before he could be taken home, Matthew, his family, and the ward staff were in something akin to a state of readiness.

Whatever was going on here, I think that until Matthew's account of his inner world of meaning was heard, acknowledged, and affirmed, until he had felt this spiritual dimension of himself to be understood, the totality of his person had not been addressed and cared for. He was suffering an additional degree of lostness. He was cut off from hope until he had marked his place in his own spiritual inner world. He was cut off from his parents in so far as the family had no acknowledged spiritual map in common.

The parents were not well placed to respond when their son raised his urgent and ultimate concerns. Their culture had not prepared them to deal easily with any religious expression of the faith which had once pervaded and vital-ized it. In the circumstances, they were not free to imagine themselves into their son's map, nor, in their pain, had they the capacity to convince him that they could understand where he was. He had moved out of their range. It was a broken deep level link in the relationship, and part of the pastoral task, if you like, the healing task, was to help its renewal.

It was difficult for his parents to work with their sense of failing Matthew at the very time when he needed to open up on his inner thoughts. Yet when they were helped to realize that he was struggling to uncover a deeper context of relationship, pushing out beyond himself into a wider continuity of existence, the bleakness of their condition was warmed, like their son's, by a kind of joy. His body was wasting, but he was not dying inside. He was making them a gift.

Such a statement may seem outrageous, as may any talk of a healing task in this context. Yet Matthew was giving his parents the means to create something new, and, in so doing, to regain a measure of control. Consciously or unconsciously, he enabled a new connectedness, a movement in their thinking away from future loss towards the deep inner present. Together, the family were putting purpose and value into something otherwise unthinkable, ensuring that this 'now', which would become 'the past' would not be lost, and that the parents could begin to live from a new place within themselves.

CONNECTIONS

The children with whom this chapter began were making connections. In the story of Matthew, the word 'connectedness' is used. What I am here calling the spiritual, as distinct from the religious (Stoter 1995) is the profound quality of ordinary human life, is sometimes seen in terms of making connections, whether with someone, a person, or a group, or with something, say, some natural phenomenon. Whether or not there is a transcendent reference, the sense of connectedness surely belongs to the whole human race, while the interpretation of that 'someone or something' will vary across cultures.

Culture has been defined as

'a set of guidelines (both explicit and implicit) which individuals inherit as members of a particular society, and which tells them how to view the world, how to experience it emotionally, and how to behave in it in relation to other people, to supernatural forces or gods, and to the natural environment . . . ' (Helman 1990.)

Once more, it is clear how spiritual and cultural are interwoven and, I think, for sensitive support of the family damaged by imminent or actual loss of a child, how crucial it is to give attention to the world of meaning. Even though Matthew, his parents, and those delivering care shared one culture, it was difficult to provide a secure, containing environment for his last moments until the spiritual had been dealt with. When cultures meet, the situation becomes more complex.

SAIRA

Saira was the months-old daughter of an English father and a mother from a Mediterranean background, who had come together after previous broken marriages. Their relationship was not accepted by their families and, as a consequence, Saira was defiantly and desperately loved. When it was clear that nothing further could be done to give her any chance of life, her parents asked to see a chaplain. If they knew why they were making this request they were unable to frame their reason in words. And if they had been able to identify and articulate anything that might be called religious belief, it would have fitted no traditional mould. Something impelled them to seek the representative of a faith community and to speak of lostness, their child's and their own.

A means of giving place and identity to the baby was devised, a ceremony by which her existence could be invested with due value and significance. This released powerful emotion and made possible some examination of the anger and guilt which the parents were feeling. They were angry about what life had brought them, angry with their parents and relatives for abandoning them, angry at 'god-if-god-exists'. Most of all, they were angry at themselves, and feeling guilty about having put themselves outside the traditions in which they had been brought up. It was as if they imagined having crossed a forbidden line and drawn punishment upon themselves and pain upon the child for whom they were responsible. It would take time for them to allow themselves a degree of forgiveness and peace. As a means towards that, we tried, when Saira died, to construct a farewell ceremony which recognized the integrity of the secular father and mother as individuals and as a couple, which affirmed their spiritual nature, and which drew on the religious expressions of that nature into which they had been born and from which they had moved, namely western Christianity and Islam. The occasion brought the wider families into a measure of contact which, it emerged, had been as desired as it had been feared. And it allowed Saira's father a voice as he said his goodbye at the graveside with difficulty and dignity.

For some time afterwards, the child's mother spoke of her daily pain and a hunger to smell Saira close to her. At the same time she manifested a new connectedness to meaning and a renewed rootedness in the relationship to her partner and to her wider family community as links, not so much broken as never made, were forged. It was not that every question had been answered for this couple, far from it. They were developing a fearlessness about facing their impotence, their sense of dependency and lingering feeling of being punished, and they were marking out these spiritual issues on a new map of their world of meaning.

TUNING IN

The families of Matthew and of Saira were each, as it were, redrawing the outline of the hand, each going through a transformation of self-definition, of priorities, maybe even of value. Sensitivity to this spiritual process required careful listening on the helper's part and a willingness to let go of presuppositions about categories and labels. Such willingness is necessary when meeting people of any of the fabulous and varied cultural backgrounds in British society today. Place of birth, education, lifestyle, these will be among the factors in play, as will religion. But belief systems are complex and subtle. Customs and practices within them differ from family to family, from individual to individual. There is no one Christianity. It seems unlikely that there is only one Judaism, one Buddhism. No tradition is to be reduced to a few sentences in a handbook, and the health worker must be prepared to live with the discomfort of feeling de-skilled and inadequate, to learn to let the family show the way. However, there is value in having an idea of some of the spiritual signposts which may guide the steps of men and women in crisis and loss. The following paragraphs are offered with a view to enabling some recognition of what might be required for care to be attuned to the family's world of meaning.

The Buddhist community

Within the three main movements of Buddhism, there is a great diversity of culturally conditioned practice. Each follower, however, is conscious of looking back to, and walking in the path of, the Indian teacher entitled Buddha. The path guides attitudes, conduct, and thought with a view to liberating the follower from the cycle of rebirth in which all living things are caught. Nothing is permanent. Unhappiness, dissatisfaction, suffering, these are only to be expected as realities of life. And so, the mind is conditioned through meditation to accept with serenity whatever comes.

The Buddhist family would hope to face the loss of a child with quietness and calm acceptance. All that encourages them in this is likely to be appreciated. There is no minister of religion with a pastoral role at this time, but a visit from a Buddhist monk or sister of the appropriate school might be welcome. When the child dies, there are no specific rituals, though, again, a monk's presence might be valued and some candles welcome to enable contemplation and a serene farewell. There are no formal constraints as to who may touch the body. Refusal of a request for a post-mortem would be unlikely. The lunar calendar governs the timing of the funeral, and the family culture, the method of disposal. A wake might be held, and the anniversary of death observed thereafter.

The Christian community

Here too, we find three main movements in the form of churches: Orthodox, Catholic, and Protestant; a multiplicity of forms and a matrix of creative tensions, rather than agreed truth. However, at the centre of the Christian map of meaning is the idea of the divine reaching into, and providing a model for, human living in the figure of Jesus. The drama of salvation, recounted in scripture, portrayed in liturgy, is a source of strength to followers of this way. Whether devout or detached, the Christian family facing the loss of a child, may find compelling support in the hope of a life to come and a gospel which connects with helplessness, abandonment, and grieving.

In most Christian groups, ordained ministers have a recognized pastoral role and, at such a time, will be ready to bring the resources of their community of faith to bear. These may range through sacramental use of oil or water, prayer with varying intention, scripture and other devotional reading. The emphasis within each church will not be the same, so the denominational label owned by the family should be taken into account. Roman Catholics and Orthodox, for example, would be likely to look for priestly ministration with a set form, while for Free Church members an informal blend of scripture and prayer would be more meaningful. Whatever the practice, and this would apply also to religious traditions beyond the Christian one, the aim would be to help contain the deepest feelings in confrontation with suffering and death, to locate the family in the context of wider loving support, and to provide a measure of peace in their inner uproar.

In the Christian mainstream, no religious considerations govern attitudes to post-mortem requests, laying out the body, or choice of burial or cremation.

The Hindu community

Teeming imagination characterizes the Hindu world of meaning which finds expression in rich devotional writing and practice, and gives religious sanction to striking social arrangements. It is permeated by myriad gods and spirits, all of them manifestations of one reality, the Supreme Being, whose existence is reflected in every person and in every living thing. All levels of life are bound together in a continuing flux of birth and rebirth, the divine will being that through conduct in this life, the conditions of the next life are formed. So liberation from the cycle of rebirth may be accelerated or retarded, but ultimately the progression will be through tribulation to final bliss. Even so, when a Hindu family face the loss of a child, it can be difficult to ascertain whether their apparent equanimity is born of assurance or fatalism.

In such circumstances, home, where most Hindu religious activity takes place, would be the preferred context. Whether there or in hospital, health workers could find any or all of the following being carried out to help the child's next life: prayers, reading of holy scripture, the tying of thread in blessing, the use of holy water, and other religious symbols. The family might want the child's body to be laid on the floor to be closer to earth and they might value the presence of the pandit, priest, as these observances were being carried out. In hospital, the prayers of a chaplain might be sought. Hindus are usually tolerant of other outlooks, and no one should fear making gentle enquiries about their expectations.

At the time of death and after, it should be borne in mind that, though unlikely to be refused, a request for a post-mortem might not be welcome. The family would hope for the speedy release of the child so as to prepare for disposal as soon as possible. They might want to perform last offices themselves, in which case the body should be wrapped in a plain sheet with threads or jewellery left in place to await attention. Or it could be acceptable for the health worker to wash the body, perhaps wearing disposable gloves to avoid causing possible later distress. Though Hindus follow a practice of cremation, younger children are more usually buried. A mourning period is observed and a remembrance ceremony may be held on the anniversary of the death.

The Jewish community

The Jewish journey has been long, determined, and heroic. Exile and dispersion, suffering and survival, these are its tokens. In this world of meaning, history and faith beget an identity seen in the community's covenant with the single all-creating deity who, through Moses, gave a framework for living, known as the Torah. Sabbath by Sabbath, the Torah is read in synagogue and its precepts carried out in worship of God and in ethical living. The homeliness and majesty of this religion combine to cradle the Jewish family confronting the death of a child. Friends may gather to say prayers and psalms and, whether the family are orthodox, reform, or liberal, a rabbi may be of much comfort and counsel.

Upon the death of the child, a family member may gently close the eyes and mouth, and lay the arms straight by the sides. The jaw may be bound, and the body placed in a plain sheet, sometimes laid on the floor with a candle at the head. If no family can be present, it may be permissible for hospital staff to carry out these procedures, preferably using disposable gloves and moving the body to the mortuary. What should not happen, however, is for the body to be washed or be left unattended. It may be that a watcher will keep vigil until the time of burial which is normally within twenty-four hours unless the Sabbath or a festival intervenes. The orthodox will resist any request for a post-mortem and insist upon burial in a Jewish cemetery after ritual purification. A more flexible approach will perhaps characterize others, but all will be likely to meet the reality of death head on, and to encourage open expression of grief at the funeral. Over the following year, a formal pattern of mourning will provide the bereaved with the support of their community.

The Muslim community

Drawn from many and varied races, this community is given unity and cohesion by a map of meaning which differentiates clearly between the road to hell and the path to paradise. They are Muslim who are faithful, and it is uncompromising faithfulness to the law of the one and only god which will bring them to him. That law, which was revealed by God to Muhammad his prophet, is contained in one book the Qur'an, in one language, Arabic. Islam, at once a creed, political system, and social order, makes five fundamental demands. First is the confession of faith that Allah is the one true god and that Muhammad is his prophet. The second is for daily prayer in accordance with the prescribed manner and time, joining others at the mosque on Fridays. The third is for observance of the annual fast. Regular giving of alms to the poor is fourth, and the fifth is for a once in a lifetime pilgrimage to Mecca when circumstances permit.

There are competing trends, movements, and cultural variations within Islam, but it is probably to be expected that the loss of a child will be seen as in some way happening within the will of Allah. Resignation may characterize the family members whose faith will require that they pray at this time, perhaps aloud, perhaps in the ear of the child. If in hospital, all that can be done to facilitate prayer by way of space, access to water, and privacy will be appreciated. The imam, who is a leader of prayer in the mosque rather than a pastor, has no specific role here, but reference to his availability might be important. The family may be grateful if the child's bed can be turned with its foot in the direction of Mecca. When death comes, grief may be loud, though some may want to suppress emotion as a sign of faith and surrender. Words of faith will be spoken, 'Surely we are Allah's and to him we shall surely return.'

The requirement is then for the health worker, wearing disposable gloves, to straighten the body, close mouth and eyes, turn the head toward the right shoulder, and fasten the great toes together. The child should not be washed, but, complete with religious jewellery, wrapped in a plain white sheet to await last offices performed by a relative. Burial in the homeland is the ideal. Burial as soon after death as possible is the necessity. A post-mortem examination is not generally acceptable unless there is legal requirement, in which case it is important to assure the family that organs removed will be returned to the body for burial. Duty binds friends and relatives to a supportive programme of mourning, and anniversary remembrances remain important.

One final point should be noted. If a mother loses her child within forty days of delivery, any encouragement to hold her baby should be tentative, tempered by the knowledge that, strictly speaking, her faith forbids the touching of a dead body.

The Sikh community

The religion of the Sikhs may be seen as emerging from the encounter between Islam and Hinduism in a particular time and place. A reform movement, building on the devotional current within Hinduism and the disciplined prayer and monotheism of Islam, it attempted a synthesis of the two. But the dream of Nanak and the other Gurus failed. Persecution forged the disciplines of this way into a separate community identifying themselves by five marks which remain of religious significance to this day. They are, hair that is uncut, a comb for holding the hair, white undershorts worn at all times, a small dagger, and a steel bangle. In this map of meaning, the way to liberation from the cycle of rebirth to union with God is by the living of a good life, showing kindness and concern to others. The Gurdwara is the temple where religious and social activities take place. Here, the Sikh child is named and later taken for baptism. Here, prayer ceremonies are held every day, the holy book, Guru Granth Sahib, being the focus of devotion.

It is in reading from this holy book and from mutual solidarity that comfort may come as Sikh family members gather to contend with the loss of a child. If they are present at the time of death, the family may show the way by normally wanting to wash and dress the body themselves. The health worker may lay the child flat, straightening limbs and closing eyes, then, without disturbing any of the symbols of Sikhism, wrap the body in a plain white sheet. Though the idea of a post-mortem is not liked, no religious objection is usually offered. Cremation follows within twenty-four hours if possible, the coffin having gone for prayers to the home and sometimes to the Gurdwara. Official mourning then binds the whole family at home for a period within which the wider community visit to pay their respects.

CODA

'To acquire information is not to be bitten by reality' says the theologian (Williams 1972). Rarely is this more true than when faced with a family in the process of losing a child, we flee to the appropriate section of a chapter like this. And what of the galaxy of cultural and spiritual values untouched in these pages? My purpose throughout has been not so much to give information, of which no book could contain enough in the first place, but to emphasize the beckoning nature of the child and of human selfhood, and to underline the possibility of the knowing that is a kind of communion. Such possibility both poses threat and hones the edge of this work. Yet it is openness to such possibility that will alone break down isolation, and release whatever it is that we call support.

'All these things entered you as if they were both the door and what came through it. They marked the spot, marked time and held it open' (Heaney 1991). We cannot, from the outside, pretend to know the deep and permanent trace which such an experience will leave on the map of meaning of a particular family. We can, however, begin to recognize and acknowledge its crucial nature in a way that allows us to stay within reach of the family as they begin to cut their path through loss and earn their own peace.

REFERENCES

Clark, J. (1991). From the lap of the Gods . . . into our own hands. *Sea of Faith Magazine*, 7, 12.

Heaney, S. (1991). From markings. In *Seeing things*, p. 9. Faber, London.

Helman, C. G. (1990). *Culture, health and illness*, p. 2. Wright, London.

Stoter, D. (1995). *Spiritual aspects of health care*. Mosby, London.

Williams, H. (1972). *True resurrection*, p. 66. Mitchell Beazley, London.

Winnicott, D. (1965). *The family and individual development*, p. 43. Tavistock, London.

9

Bereavement

Dora Black

INTRODUCTION

Palliation is not cure, and death must ensue in due course. This chapter considers the effect a child's death has on those left behind—the parents, siblings, and others close to the child and family (friends, relatives, teachers, nursing, and medical staff). It outlines normal grieving patterns in adults and children of different ages, and what can be done to help progress through the normal, but often painful experience of mourning. The mourning process may become pathological and we shall look at the various patterns, and what treatments can help. Finally, the prevention of pathological outcomes is addressed and how children and young people can be prepared for the effects of loss and bereavement as part of their general education.

NORMAL PARENTAL GRIEF

From the moment a child is born, a process of mutual parent–child attachment begins (Bowlby 1969). This process, which is biologically determined and which occurs in all higher mammals, serves an important function to aid survival in species where a long period of immaturity occurs. When that bond is disrupted, grief follows. Hinde (1979) has described grief reactions to loss in primates which exactly match those in humans. Parkes (1986) has described in detail the phenomenology of adult grief after the death of a spouse, and the evidence is that these experiences are universal (Rosenblatt *et al*. 1976). Immediately after the death of someone to whom we are attached, we react with disbelief and denial.

'It can't be true' or 'It hasn't happened!' are common responses to such devastating news. However, the evidence of one's eyes cannot long be denied and the second, 'protest' phase of grief begins, characterized by crying loudly (or wailing), motor restlessness, and agitation. When frantic efforts to wake the dead are unsuccessful, the bereaved parent moves into the third phase of grief when the death is acknowledged and mourning begins. This phase resembles an acute depressive illness. If we did not know that bereavement had occurred, we might diagnose depression. Movements are slowed (psychomotor retardation), crying becomes quieter and sadder (keening), self-reproaches are common. 'If only we hadn't agreed to the bone marrow transplant' or 'If we had taken him to be treated by the faith healer', etc. Anger can be a troubling emotion at this time but it is not universal. Finally, some kind of adaptation to the loss occurs in normal grief and life without the dead child can continue. This final phase may not come for many months and requires a considerable amount of 'grief work' (Freud 1917) to be done to move from being the parent of an ill but alive child, to perhaps (in the case of an only child) not being a parent at all, or being the parent of a baby but not a toddler any more, etc. Bowlby and Parkes (1970) suggest that the first two phases of grief have a protective function in that they enable the human psyche to have a respite from the duties and responsibilities of normal life to enable the grief work to be done, which aids adaptation after a loss. Denial gives the psyche time to take in the magnitude of the news for which it may not be prepared, whilst the hyperactivity of the 'protest' phase enables the lost one to be found if he or she has not died but merely strayed from sight.

THE COURSE OF MOURNING

Progress through the phases of grief is not straightforward or only in one direction. But in normal grief, there is a discernible movement forward over time. Denial does not persist when the bereaved parent is confronted with the reality of the body of his or her dead child, and it is helpful therefore both to see and to touch the dead child even though the attempts made to 'wake the dead' might be distressing to the onlooker who is unfamiliar with death. Western culture tends to discourage the expression and display of extreme emotion, although there is evidence that it is helpful in promoting progress through the phases of grief, and promoting mental recovery (Parkes 1986). Many other cultures have ritualized their mourning practices and it is essential for nurses and doctors working in a multicultural society to be familiar with the mourning rituals of the various ethnic groups in their area (see Chapter 8).

When the depressive phase ensues, the parent may slip back into excesses of agitated crying and searching, wringing his or her hands, running around calling for the dead child, and visiting haunts where the child used to be. Each of these searches results in failure and the sadness, crying, and the realization of the permanence of the loss wells up again and again. It seems that, to be enabled to move from one 'assumptive world' as Parkes (1971) has called it, to another, we have to experience repeatedly the reality of loss. The depressive phase of grief is a very painful one. The parent reviews his or her life with the child and may go over in his or her mind the things done wrongly, or the omissions that may have made a difference. Self-reproach and suicidal thoughts are not uncommon.

Even when the parent has moved on and found some way of living without the dead child and has resumed many of the normal daily activities, a chance reminder of the dead child may plunge the parent back into depression again. Sometimes the emotion precedes the consciousness of the reminder. A tune the child sang often, or a favourite toy in another's hands may cause renewed pangs of grief and floods of tears, and yet the parent may be unconscious of the actual trigger at first, so the sudden emotion is startling to the parent as well as the onlooker.

DURATION OF MOURNING

The progress of the phases of grief is not uniform. The duration depends on the closeness of the relationship, the preparation for the death, and the appropriateness of it. The grieving process is most straightforward after the death of elderly parents when they have had a short but clearly terminal illness, and when the survivors have separated physically. Conversely, grief is longer when the death is sudden, unexpected, and untimely. Most children's deaths are untimely, and many of them are sudden, and for the parents at least, unexpected.

In a normal grief reaction, the acute pangs of grief last a few weeks or months at the most, the depressive phase can also go on for some months, and by the first, or at most the second anniversary, there is considerable improvement. However, many parents feel that they never really recover from the loss of a child. They may adjust to it, they may be able to resume their everyday activities, and may even derive some pleasure from life, but they feel they remain vulnerable, and they are not the same people they were before (Osterweis *et al.* 1984). For some parents, the new identity is a stronger one—they feel they have been 'through the fire' and that nothing can affect them so profoundly again. The cost may be loss of sensitivity to their other children or their partner, which may threaten the marriage or even disrupt it.

PATHOLOGICAL GRIEF REACTIONS IN PARENTS

Recovery from grief can only occur when the reality of the loss has been accepted, the pain of grief has been experienced, the bereaved parent has adjusted to the environment in which the dead child is no longer there, and that parent has withdrawn the emotional investment in that child to invest in another relationship (Worden 1982). For bereaved parents these tasks are particularly difficult. Bereaved parents can often deny the reality of the loss of a child, unlike that of a spouse because of the presence of other children. Their continuing need for care both prevents a parent from mourning and enables them to deny the need for it. If the child who dies is an infant, society too may deny the reality of the parental role. 'You hardly had time to get to know him' or 'you must be thankful that it wasn't one of the older children' are commonly heard by parents who lose young children. For these and other reasons, parental bereavement is unlike other forms of bereavement (Rando 1986) and carries a higher risk of pathology. One recent study of parental reactions following sudden death found that over 70 per cent of parents experienced intense and troubling grief reactions especially if the child was over one year in age, and in one third of the cases the marriage deteriorated (Sumner and Dinwiddie 1989).

Absent, delayed, prolonged, or distorted grief

These pathological bereavement reactions occur more commonly when the loss is sudden, unexpected, untimely, or horrific (mutilation, etc.), when there have been deaths preceding or following, and where social supports are lacking (Parkes 1985).

Hussein, aged 11, died suddenly after vomiting blood and developing a convulsion, following a bone marrow transplant for acute lymphoblastic leukaemia. He came from abroad for treatment and his parents lacked family here, and even a language in common with the staff of the hospital who were themselves traumatized by the sudden and horrific nature of the death. The parents became frozen in their reaction. For the time they remained in this country, they refused to accept that Hussein had died. The mother continued to come to the ward and to visit the room he had inhabited, becoming angry that another child now had taken his place. When they returned to their home, their relatives were concerned at the absence of grief, which in that country was usually openly displayed.

If grief reactions are delayed, society initially mobilized by the death to support the family, fades away so that the bereaved person, when grief comes in, grieves alone. Similarly, if the parent continues to grieve after the time that his friends and family feel he should have 'got over it', they will melt away, and he will be unsupported. Both these forms of grief lead to a higher incidence of psychological and physical dysfunction.

Distorted grief reactions include exaggerated forms of normal grief—such as excessive guilt, or anger. These occur more commonly in parents. Parents are responsible for protecting their children and death is seen as the ultimate failure to protect and rear. One way of dealing with the pain of guilt is to use a projective defence mechanism and intensely angry feelings may be directed towards doctors, the hospital, and sometimes, their partner or the siblings.

One way of coping with the death of a child is by idealization or mummification. The latter refers to the habit of freezing the room, possessions, and image of the lost child. No one is allowed to use his things. His or her clothes are not handed on and a shrine is created. If the child is also idealized, the burden for the remaining siblings may be too great. Visiting the cemetery daily or weekly may use up scarce physical and emotional energy, and prove costly. One study of children who had died from cystic fibrosis found that most parents had preserved the child's room as a shrine or had visited the grave at least weekly, more than a year after the death (Kerner *et al.* 1979).

Another unique parental reaction to the loss of a child is to wish for a replacement child (Cain and Cain 1964). Most authorities suggest that embarking on another pregnancy before a period of mourning has been completed enhances the likelihood that the new child will have difficulties in establishing an identity that is distinct from the dead child (Pine and Brauer 1986).

There is some evidence that the place of death has an influence on the course of mourning. Mulhern and colleagues (1983), for example found that parents were more anxious, depressed, and defensive after death in hospital than at home, and Lauer *et al.* (1989) found that when children died at home, the long-term outcome was better for the parents.

One of the problems in evaluating the research on bereaved parents is it often fails to control for the length of the preceding illness. On the one hand, grief is more difficult after a sudden unexpected death and a prolonged illness can provide the family with definite knowledge of the impending death and the opportunity for anticipatory mourning. On the other hand, since life-threatening illness in children affects family functioning adversely in a large proportion of cases, the parents and siblings may be starting their bereavement from an already disturbed or distressed state of mind. Maguire's (1983) controlled study found that after diagnosis of leukaemia in a child, one third of the mothers were suffering from an anxiety state and one third from depression, and 12–18 months later, a quarter of the mothers were suffering from each of these conditions. There was also a substantial deterioration in sexual adjustment during the course of the illness. Few of these mothers had sought or had any help for these problems and indeed, another study found that family doctors rarely enquired about family functioning when a child is sick (Rosser and Maguire 1982).

High rates of morbidity after death are more likely when there has been pre-bereavement psychological ill health, and as we have seen, this correlates with the length of the illness prior to death (Rando 1983).

THE EFFECT ON CHILDREN OF THE DEATH OF A SIBLING

The way a child reacts to death will be determined by his or her age and understanding of death, the prior relationship with the sibling, how he or she has been prepared, and how the parents deal with their own grief.

Understanding of death

Young children are as intelligent as older ones but they lack experience and knowledge. They will struggle to comprehend what is happening and will fantasize in the absence of an explanation. A most helpful description of a 3-year-old's attempt to grapple with his sister's death is to be found in Fabian (1988). It is clear from this account and others that even very young children can be helped to understand that death is permanent, irreversible, happens to everyone, has a cause, and that dead people differ from live people in a number of respects (see Chapter 5). Because of their ego-centricity and their animistic view of the world, children may believe that they have caused an event if they wished it or did something wrong.

When Judith died of Graft versus Host disease after a bone marrow transplant from her seven-year-old brother Jim, he became very disturbed, waking three or four times a night and crying inconsol-ably. Sensitive questioning by a therapist enabled him to express his belief that his marrow had killed his sister. In a sense, of course it had and he had overheard conversations to that effect. He needed to be helped to understand that because his marrow was not of help to Judith, he had not himself wanted to kill her or been the cause of her death—it was the disease itself which she had not been able to throw off.

As children mature, so does their understanding of death. There is no doubt that it is possible to help most children of normal intelligence and many mentally retarded children to understand the concepts outlined above. What causes many misconceptions is the failure of adults to help the child with an explanation that is appropriate to his stage of develop-ment. The child often has to struggle to make sense of stories which do not make sense. Daniel, at three (Fabian 1988), was told that sister Sarah had gone to the angels. Later, his mother regretted this as she saw his struggles to cope with this story that did not fit in with anything else he was experiencing or perceiving, or that his parents believed.

Processes of grief in children

Can children grieve? For years, there was controversy about whether children could relinquish attachment to a parent because of their continuing need for parenting. Wolfenstein (1966), for example, considered that mourning could not take place before adolescence. Bowlby (1969), in his monumental work *Attachment and loss*, reviewed all the literature and came to the conclusion that whilst it was possible for children of almost any age to go through the stages of mourning identified in adults, there was a much greater risk of pathological mourning reactions in children because of limitations in their understanding and in what they have been allowed to know. Those working with bereaved children have found that, with help, children as young as four or five can be helped to understand that the death is permanent and irreversible, and be helped to mourn the loss.

The first stage of grief, denial, may be prolonged in children because they are not given an opportunity to comprehend the reality. Children are often not allowed to visit, to see the sick child, or to take part in helping to care for him or her. They do not see the child after death, and often do not go to the funeral.

It is possible for children to miss the absent sibling and to enter into a state of depression when they realize that he or she is not going to return.

Joan, aged 11, was present when her seven-year-old brother, to whom she was devoted, was run over and killed. She was able to join in the family grief, and in family therapy sessions to talk about her loneliness now she was an only child. She had no one to share the joys and sorrows of childhood with, she felt. She mourned the fights they could no longer have and eventually she persuaded her parents to have another child!

Relationship with sibling

Siblings show rivalry for parental attention. Dunn *et al.* (1981) have shown that the greatest trauma that many young children experience is the birth of a sibling with whom they have to share the hitherto exclusive attention of their parents. For the sibling of a sick child, their envy is enormous because they have lost the fight. Often they lose the parent entirely; physically, when the child takes up residence in a distant hospital, then emotionally when he or she withdraws in grief or depression, or becomes unreasonably or persistently irritable.

Children who lose a sibling have been less studied than those bereaved of a parent. Pettle Michael and Lansdown's (1986) study of 28 children found that two or three years after the death a high proportion of the children were emotionally or behaviourally disturbed and had a low self-esteem. The dead sibling was idealized, school-work suffered. If the child had been prepared, had participated in the patient's care, and had been able to take leave of him or her and joined in the community rituals, the outcome appeared better. Interestingly, their study found no correlation between parental and child adaptation. Siblings are rarely adequately prepared for death. In Rosenheim and Reicher's (1985) study of parental death, children who were informed about the death had lower levels of anxiety than those who were not, even within families. Their pre-bereavement morbidity is high. Maguire's (1983) study found that a third of the siblings of children with leukaemia developed behavioural problems, and others have found even higher rates (Peck 1979 and Cairns *et al*. 1979). About a quarter of siblings have academic and behavioural problems at school even before the death (Eiser 1980). Children are more likely than adults to develop pathological mourning reactions.

EFFECTS OF THE DEATH OF A CHILD ON OTHERS

Family

Grandparents are often involved as carers for the other children and supports for the parents. They rarely are included in any support provided by the hospital and no studies have been done of their reactions. Because they usually have to learn about the illness, and prognosis at second-hand, they may be bewildered and can be obstructive. They may encourage fruitless and expensive searches for alternative treatments. Other relatives may be similarly in the dark, while carrying a burden of support and care. Their grief reactions need acknowledgement.

The community

Others in the world of the family and the child, friends, teachers, and neighbours, are caught up in the tragedy of the death and may be able to be very helpful to the family but their own grief may not have been acknowledged and worked through. There is a place for a community mourning ritual which is usually the funeral or the memorial service. It is important that bereaved parents are helped to see the usefulness of a public community ritual.

Friends of the child are often denied recognition of their loss. They are given even less information than adults, and because of their immaturity are not able to comprehend what is being discussed over their head. Rituals such as that described by Arngrimmson (1984) conducted at school or by a club can be therapeutic.

Professional staff

Those doctors, nurses, teachers, and other professionals caring for a child who dies are themselves bereaved. They may have known the child for many years and have come to love her or him. It is important that the senior members of the team acknowledge this and support their staff through their own grief. The dangers of neglecting this are that the individual may develop maladaptive psychological defences or give so much of themselves that they burn out (Raphael 1982). The rewards of caring for dying children are immense but they have to be recognized (Dominica 1987) and those in charge must ensure rest periods and an opportunity to work through the grief of the staff, through group meetings with a leader who has skill and knowledge in bereavement counselling. Many wards find it helpful to have a meeting following a death and use it to review their contact with the dead child and the joys and sorrows of their relationship. It is important for those less closely associated with the child and family to express condolences to the staff nearest the child. In this way, it is acknowledged that feelings matter and a ward ethos develops which gives due regard to their importance.

INTERVENTION TECHNIQUES

There is now good evidence that many of the pathological grief reactions outlined above can be prevented or modified by intervention, either before the death when possible, or during the period following death. Parkes (1980) in a review of controlled studies of the efficacy of bereavement counselling for adults, concluded that it was helpful, and Black and Urbanowicz's (1984) controlled trial of family therapy with children bereaved of a parent, showed that the post-bereavement morbidity of 50 per cent at one year, could be reduced to 20 per cent by six sessions of family meetings which focused on promoting shared grief and mourning within the family, and encouraging communication about the dead parent. Furman and her colleagues' sensitive work with individual children, whilst not controlled, gives pointers to the problems that bereavement poses for children and how they can be helped (Furman 1974).

WHO SHOULD PROVIDE PSYCHOSOCIAL SUPPORT AND HELP

Many paediatricians and nurses spend much of their time in spiritual and psychological care of their patients and their relatives (Burton 1974, Dominica 1987). However, the sole formally trained psychosocial professional available in many departments is a social worker. In addition to their knowledge of benefits and charitable funds available to the families, most social workers have a training in one or more of the therapeutic techniques mentioned above. It is unlikely, however, that one person can embody all the therapeutic techniques available for helping these families, and one study of the efficacy of social work help was disappointing in finding no differences between the probands and controls in outcome on a number of variables (Nolan *et al.* 1987). Chaplains, particularly in hospital, have an important counselling role

with many patients and families, not only those of their
religious faith (Speck 1978). Their contribution has not been
evaluated.

Ideally, every family should receive good quality psychosocial support and counselling before and after the death.
Any paediatric service which is treating terminally ill children should have access to a wide range of psychological
services for the children and their families, including
psychology, psychiatry, and psychotherapy (individual,
family, and behavioural). A routine involvement avoids
creating the feeling in an already stressed family, that the
paediatrician thinks that they are 'mad' or that they are
singular in needing such help.

Family therapy and parental counselling may be the preventative interventions of choice before and after bereavement; we await controlled studies. The tasks of the therapist
or counsellor before death can be summarized as follows:

(1) to ascertain what is known, what is understood, who
    knows and understands it;

(2) to address child-care issues;

(3) to help cope with the psychological effects of the diag-
    nosis, illness, and treatment on patient and family;

(4) to help with treatment compliance;

(5) to address issues of intimacy;

(6) to enhance the patient's feeling of autonomy and
    mastery;

(7) to help with family cohesion and communication;

(8) to help patient and family adjust to limitations imposed
    by the disease and its treatment;

(9) to help families cope with the family change;

(10) to help patient and family to address issues of death and
    dying, and to face death.

The tasks during and after death include the most difficult one for doctors, nurses, chaplains, counsellors, and
therapists of *being* with, rather than *doing* anything. What
families appreciate most is the presence of someone they

know and trust who is not discomforted by being in the presence of death and dying, and can share their sadness and grief.

After death, the bereaved generally appreciate being supported by those with whom they are familiar. Bereavement counselling can help promote and resolve grief and mourning, and there is now good evidence from a number of research studies that counselling can prevent morbid grief reactions in adults, especially those in the high risk categories (Parkes 1980).

After Rosine's death from leukaemia, her parents' grief reactions were monitored by the psychiatric team who had been closely involved with counselling the family before death. They were grateful to the staff for the easy death of their daughter who had slipped peacefully away with her parents by her side, and they seemed to be able to express their grief normally and to gain comfort from a loving family and community. No specific intervention was needed until the father died suddenly of a heart attack after a short illness which was handled badly by the hospital concerned. The effect of the two deaths in quick succession, the sudden unexpected nature of the father's death and the mismanagement, combined to put mother in the high risk category for pathological grief. The child psychiatrist used techniques described by Raphael (1982). Mother was encouraged gently to review her life with her husband and to remember the good and bad times. Each memory was grieved for, one at a time. She would never be able to go to see her homeland again with him, nor to share the joy of their grandchildren with him, or the sorrows of their loss of Rosine, etc. At each grief the therapist forced the mother to cry and to imagine a life without her partner. This work was painful and took many sessions. After a few months, mother began to take more interest in the rest of her family, and when she decided to take driving lessons in father's car, which had stood in the garage since his death, the corner seemed to be turned. Every year after that on the anniversary of Rosine's death and again on father's, the therapist offered a meeting (see Renvoise and Jain 1986). This was accepted for the first two years, but the third year it seemed unnecessary to the mother.

Preventative intervention can also be used with siblings, who are in a high risk category. Family therapy techniques seem pragmatically to be economical, feasible, and effective but have not been evaluated when a sibling dies. As well as encouraging the child to talk about and grieve for her or his sibling, ensuring that they have understood what has happened, and that it was not their fault is essential. To help with understanding, it may be helpful to view the body and attend the funeral (Cathcart 1988; Weller *et al.* 1988). When children develop morbid grief reactions, brief interventions may not be sufficient to prevent later pathology.

When Gloria's older sister died, she couldn't stop crying. Her grief never seemed to end. A year later, when she was 11, her parents sought help from a family therapist. A brief intervention seemed effective—Gloria was able to acknowledge that she thought that inheriting her sister's toys and room felt as if she had somehow been glad of her death. This recognition helped her to recover from her chronic grief, especially when her parents' reaction was not one of blame but of understanding. However, five years' later, when under stress from examinations, she became severely depressed and took an overdose of drugs prescribed for her depression.

Techniques available include individual, family, and group meetings. These latter are usefully run at the hospital where the child died but some self-help societies offer individual and group counselling which may be more appropriate when the child died at home, if the hospital is at a distance, or when there is a reluctance to return there. Parents often appreciate the opportunity to meet with other bereaved parents (see Appendix B). Newton *et al.* (1986) and Brent (1983) have described their practices as physicians in meeting parents after a death. When pathological reactions occur such as school phobia (Black 1974), or depression in later childhood, the treatment needs to include an attempt to force mourning using appropriate techniques for the age of the child. These would include drawing, modelling, the use of dolls and animals to represent family members, and psychotherapy. The reader is referred to Rutter *et al.* (1994) for a fuller account of therapeutic techniques in child psychiatry.

PREPARATION FOR LOSS

Can we better prepare children and young people for the inevitable small losses of their lives and will this enhance their coping capacities when bigger losses occur? The first funeral a child attends should not have to be that of his sibling. Should they not be included in the grief of their community as happens in other cultures? So that when a neighbour or a community elder dies, the children attend the funeral or memorial service. If we encouraged parents to prepare their children for the possibility of loss by, for example taking the opportunity to talk about the inevitable small losses of childhood and helping them to express their grief and accept comfort, and if the opportunity was taken while visiting a church to wander round the tombstones and ponder on the lives of those buried, natural discussion of death and dying, and its effects would arise.

Recently, two manuals for teachers have been published which help to teach about the ubiquity of death and the way in which children can help their friends who may suffer loss. The authors include a useful and full list of children's fiction which deals with issues of death and grief (Ward and Associates 1993). Most children's libraries will help with recommending fiction that may help prepare children, and some issue lists of books.

When death is near, this educational and preparational work needs to be intensified. Teachers can be very helpful in preparing the class for the impending death of one of their members, and the teachers of the siblings need also to be alerted. They may be appropriate people to accompany a bereaved child to the funeral. The bereaved parents can then feel able to give themselves up to their grief, knowing that the children have someone they know who is less affected by the death, to care for them.

'All who live must die' (*Hamlet*). The death of a child is the most poignant and painful death for all who know him or her. Yet it is possible for the family to continue to function and develop. The professional staff involved with the family at the time of the death can enhance the chances of good outcome by their care.

REFERENCES

Arngrimmson, B. (1984). A community crisis resolved by a mourning ritual. *Bereavement Care*, **3**, 18–19.

Black, D. (1974). What happens to bereaved children? *Therapeutic Education*, **2**, 15–20.

Black, D. and Urbanowicz, M. A. (1984). Bereaved children; family intervention. In *Recent research in developmental psychopathology*, (ed. Stevenson J.). JCPP Book Suppl. No. 4, Pergamon Press, Oxford.

Bowlby, J. (1969). *Attachment and loss*, Vol. 1. Hogarth, London.

Bowlby, J. and Parkes, C. M. (1970). Separation and loss within the family. In *The Child in his family*. (ed. C. J. Anthoney and C. Koupernik). Wiley, New York.

Brent, D. (1983). A death in the family; the paediatrician's role. *Pediatrics*, **72**, 645–51.

Burton, L. (ed.) (1974). *Care of the child facing death*. RKP, London.

Cain, A. C. and Cain, B. S. (1964). On replacing a child. *Journal of the American Academy of Child Psychiatry*, **3**, 443–56.

Cairns, N. U., Clark, G. M., Smith, S. D., and Lansky, S. B. (1979). Adaptation of siblings to childhood malignancy. *Journal of Pediatrics*, **95**, 485–7.

Cathcart, F. (1988). Seeing the body after death. *British Medical Journal*, **297**, 997–8.

Dominica, F. (1987). The role of the hospice for the dying child. *British Journal of Hospital Medicine*, **38**, 334–42.

Dunn, J., Kendrick, C., and MacNamee, R. (1981). The reaction of first-born children to the birth of a sibling: mothers' reports. *Journal of Psychology and Psychiatry and Allied Disciplines*, **22**, 1–18.

Eiser, C. E. (1980). How leukaemia affects a child's schooling. *British Journal of Social and Clinical Psychology*, **19**, 365–8.

Fabian, A. (1988). *The Daniel diary*. Grafton, London.

Freud, S. (1917). *Mourning and melancholia*, Standard edition, Vol. 14. Hogarth, London.

Furman, E. (1974). *A child's parent dies*. Yale University Press, New Haven, Connecticut.

Hinde, R. A. (1979). *Towards understanding relationships*. Academic Press, London.

Kerner, J., Harvey, B., and Lewiston, N. (1979). The impact of grief: a retrospective study of family function following loss of a child with cystic fibrosis. *Journal of Chronic Diseases*, **32**, 223.

Lauer, M. E., Mulhern, R. K., Schell, M. J., and Camitta, B. M. (1989). Long-term follow-up of parental adjustment following a child's death at home or hospital. *Cancer*, **63**, 988–94.

Maguire, G. P. (1983). The psychological sequelae of childhood leukaemia. *Recent Results in Cancer Research*, **88**, 47–56.

Mulhern, R. K., Lauer, M. E., and Hoffman, R. G. (1983). Death of a child at home or in the hospital: subsequent psychological adjustment of the family. *Pediatrics*, **71**, 743–7.

Newton, R. W., Bergin, B., and Knowles, D. (1986). Parent's interview after a child's death. *Archives of Disease in Childhood*, **61**, 711–13.

Nolan, T., Zvagulis, I., and Pless, B. (1987). Controlled trial of social work in childhood chronic illness. *Lancet*, **2**, 411–15.

Osterweis, M., Solomon, F., and Green, M. (ed.) (1984). *Bereavement: reactions, consequences and care*. National Academy Press, Washington, DC.

Parkes, C. M. (1971). Psycho-social transitions: a field for study. *Social Science & Medicine*, **5**, 101–15.

Parkes, C. M. (1980). Bereavement counselling: does it work? *British Medical Journal*, **281**, 3–6.

Parkes, C. M. (1985). Bereavement. *British Journal of Psychiatry*, **146**, 11–17.

Parkes, C. M. (1986). *Bereavement: studies of grief in adult life*, (2nd edn). Penguin, Harmondsworth.

Peck, B. (1979). Effects of childhood cancer on long term survivors and their families. *British Medical Journal*, **1**, 1327–9.

Pettle Michael, S. A. and Lansdown, R. G. (1986). Adjustment to the death of a sibling. *Archives of Disease in Childhood*, **61**, 278–83.

Pine, V. R. and Brauer, C. (1986). Parental grief: a synthesis of theory, research and intervention. In *Parental loss of a child*, (ed. T. Rando). Research Press, Chicago, Illinois.

Rando, T. A. (1983). An investigation of grief and adaptation of parents whose children have died from cancer. *Journal of Pediatric Psychology*, **8**, 3–20.

Rando, T. A. (1986). Parental bereavement: an exception to the general conceptualizations of mourning. In *Parental loss of a child*, (ed. T. Rando). Research Press, Chicago, IL.

Raphael, B. (1982). *The anatomy of bereavement*. Basic Books, New York.

Renvoise, E. B. and Jain, J. (1986). Anniversary reactions. *British Journal of Psychiatry*, **148**, 322–4.

Rosenblatt, P. C., Walsh, R. P., and Jackson, D. A. (1976). *Grief and mourning in cross-cultural perspective*. HRAF Press, New Haven, Connecticut.

Rosenheim, E. and Reicher, R. (1985). Informing children about a parent's terminal illness. *Journal of Child Psychology and Psychiatry and Allied Disciplines*, **26**, 995–8.

Rosser, J. E. and Maguire, P. (1982). Dilemmas in general practice; the care of the cancer patient. *Social Science and Medicine*, **16**, 315–22.

Rutter, M., Taylor, E., and Hersov, L. (1994). *Child psychiatry, modern approaches*, (3rd edn). Blackwell, Oxford.

Speck, P. (1978). *Loss and grief in medicine*. Baillière, London.

Sumner, M. and Dinwiddie, R. (1989). Parental bereavement. *Bereavement Care*, **8**, 21.

Ward, B. and Associates (1993). *Good grief, 1 and Good grief, 2*, (2nd edn) Jessica Kingsley, London.

Weller, E. B., Weller, R. A., Fristad, M. A., Cain, S. E., and Bowes, J. M. (1988). Should children attend their parent's funeral? *Journal of the American Academy of Child and Adolescent Psychiatry*, **27**, 559–62.

Wolfenstein, M. (1966). How is mourning possible? *Psychoanalytic Study of the Child*, **21**, 93–123.

Worden, J. W. (1982). *Grief counselling and grief therapy*. Tavistock, London.

10

Caring for the carers

Alan Stein and Helen Woolley

Individuals vary widely as to how much pressure they can bear before they experience debilitating personal distress. Pressures and stressors which appear to stimulate one person to even more productive work and innovative solutions may be quite crippling for another. Recognizing this individual variation, we aim in this chapter to identify from the literature and from our own research and experience, some of the sources of pressure on staff caring for dying children and some of the ways reported as useful in dealing with, and mediating that pressure.

WHY CARE FOR THE CARER?

Some might argue that it is a peripheral luxury to spend time addressing the staff's own emotional needs when faced with the tragedy of a dying child. There is, however, increasing evidence that when stresses are ignored or denied and staff do not get appropriate support, the consequences not only for their own emotional well-being but also for patient care may be serious. Ultimately it may affect the ability of staff to remain in their jobs (Vachon and Pakes 1984; Vachon 1987; Lattanzi 1985; Woolley *et al*. 1989). The extent to which these sorts of issues may be troublesome was recently emphasized by a survey of house officers which identified a lack of adequate training in breaking bad news as one of the most serious deficiencies in their education (Dent *et al.* 1990). The very perception of such a deficiency on the part of staff is likely to amplify their feeling that they are not doing a good job.

As early as 1960, Menzies-Lyth described how nurses caring for dying and suffering patients, especially when faced with distasteful and distressing tasks far beyond what they would normally encounter, are at considerable risk of being flooded by intense and unmanageable anxiety. Nurses are confronted by a mixture of feelings—pity, compassion, love, and hate— and can find themselves resenting the very patients who arouse such strong feelings. Menzies-Lyth argues that the 'social defence system' (first described by Jacques in 1955) may actually serve to protect the nurse from anxiety, un- certainty, and even guilt—but to the detriment of the patient's care. Sometimes the nurse is moved from ward to ward, has duties split between several patients, depersonalizes patients, has an expectation of emotional detachment, and performs ritualized tasks on the ward.

Although much has changed since 1960, Maguire (1985), when observing doctors and nurses caring for terminally ill patients, described the carers' constant use of distancing tactics which prevents them getting close to their patients' psychological suffering and discourages patients from dis- closing their emotional concerns. Such behaviour involves ignoring cues from patients, inappropriate cheerfulness, giving false reassurance, and selectively attending to certain patient concerns. These tactics may serve to ensure the staff's own 'emotional survival', but are a serious barrier to the effective psychological care of the patient. Maguire suggests that staff fear their own uncontainable strong emotions, such as despair and anger, which those they care for may evoke by revealing how he or she really feels. They also worry about upsetting the patient more by open discussion.

Many authors (Maguire 1985; Vachon and Pakes 1984; Lattanzi 1985; Vachon 1987 and 1995*b*) describe some of the impact on carers, which in effect amounts to the early stages of burn-out; increasing exhaustion, aches, pains, insomnia, irritability, and social withdrawal. Staff may become resentful and indecisive, unwilling to heed colleagues' views, cynical, rigid, and resistant to change, and resort to 'gallows humour'. Extremely dedicated staff who lack outside interests and personal support away from work often have high ideals which may put them especially at risk.

In recent years, with growing awareness of the kinds of difficulties which arise in caring for dying children, the need to find a balance in the relationship between the carer, the child, and his family, and particularly to avoid distancing tactics, has been more widely recognized. This has been epitomized by the evolution of the children's hospice movement and the move towards home-care teams in order to create a setting or working structure that minimizes the 'social defence system' and allows staff to get close to patients' and families' concerns. However, in the situation where staff are encouraged to attend carefully to families' real concerns, especially if team support and consultation is weak, they need to beware of becoming overwhelmed and of over-identifying with the families' and children's problems. Staff may become enveloped and trapped in the families' stress and despair, and lose professional independence; ultimately this leaves them unable to help the family. It can be very difficult to strike a balance, but clearly the staff need to maintain an independence of feeling and judgement which does not at the same time protect them at all costs from painful emotions.

POSSIBLE SOURCES OF STRESS

The sense of powerlessness

Lattanzi (1985) pointed to the emotional stress arising from the sense of powerlessness associated with being unable to save the life of a dying child, or eliminate the pain of bereavement. This may be particularly difficult for staff who care for terminally ill children relatively infrequently. Those regularly caring for dying children may not have expectations of cure but may still feel a sense of powerlessness when they can not fulfil their goals in symptom care and support for the family.

In our own research looking at the stresses and job satis-faction experienced by a staff group working in a children's hospice, one of the main sources of stress was the sense of impotence staff felt when they were unable to relieve perceived distress, for instance, symptoms or behaviours that seemed uncontrollable. In our study, witnessing a child's physical pain or mental distress was rated by staff as a major stressor. At times it was a struggle for staff to maintain involvement without being overwhelmed and yet preserve the inner strength to live with the distress. The staff simply had to 'live alongside' and bear with the family as they struggled through these very difficult times. How-ever, where some action to relieve symptoms could be performed, this was an important contributor to staff job satisfaction.

Many hospice staff acknowledged the positive value of 'sitting it out with the family', giving whatever comfort they could while accepting their inability to turn the main tide of events. Such care, although at the time seeming a somewhat passive partnership, was frequently reported by families at a later stage (Stein and Woolley 1990) to be one of the aspects of care they most valued. The important fact was that staff did not in any way deny or turn away from what was happening and could tolerate and therefore help partner the distress.

Dealing with critical or negative responses

One of the most difficult issues for many staff to deal with is the occasional negative or critical response from families. Many families go through a grieving process after the diagnosis is made and before the child actually dies. One of the stages of grieving that is well described is that of anger (Kubler-Ross 1970). The anger felt by the families is often most easily directed against those to whom they are closest and with whom they spend most time; as such, staff are easy targets. However, it is sometimes very difficult for staff to under-stand this while they are doing their utmost to care for the dying child. Such issues may be particularly difficult for staff working largely by themselves, such as community paediatric nurses and family doctors, who may not have anybody immediate with whom to share reactions and reach the realization that the criticisms made are not personal.

Idealism and the motivation for work

Vachon (1979, 1987) points to a number of reasons why staff working with the terminally ill are particularly at risk, especially if they lack outside support and interests. If 'staff only give of themselves without in some way being replenished they will ultimately have nothing left to give'. She points to a number of reasons why this might be so. For example, she found that work with the terminally ill attracts staff with high ideals who are inherently in danger of entertaining unrealistic expectations. Many tend to have strong religious or philosophical views which may help them to cope. Diversity amongst staff at least helps to avoid a disproportionate bias towards one strongly held view. The individual need to serve is useful in terms of the service on offer, but members of staff can find themselves debilitated if they fail to be realistic about their commitments.

Dealing with grief

Staff need time and space to talk over a death or the distressing situations they witness as part of their everyday work. They may need a place at work where they can grieve privately as well as with the parents. When a child dies, staff too need parting rituals, a chance to take their leave. Furthermore, attendance at funerals can be invaluable both as a symbol of solidarity with the family and in assisting staff with their own grief.

Grief reactions or unrecognized depression can develop in the case of long serving staff who have experienced constant confrontation with death. Initial worry or sadness in response to deaths may have developed over time into an anxiety state or depressive illness. Depression may manifest itself in poor concentration, fatigue, lack of interest in life, and sleep disturbance. Regular contact with death can also diminish ordinary relationships and have an adverse effect on friendship, marriage, and family life. There is also a danger that young or new staff with no experience of death may be quite overwhelmed by it.

In our own study, a small but distinct sub-group of staff who manifested symptoms of psychological distress were distinguished by having experienced relatively recent bereavement in their personal lives, or by having failed to resolve their grief about a bereavement which had occurred some considerable time before. Deep distress can be rekindled when a trigger event echoes back to and resurrects a sense of personal loss. Specific consideration and support needs to be given to staff who experience current personal bereavement. The very nature of the work serves as a constant reminder of their loss and may interfere with their own natural grieving. Counselling and some additional time off may be necessary.

Vachon (1987) points out that 'the professional who deals with feelings of helplessness and grief by excessive intellectualisation, flight into activity, denial, rationalisation, and withdrawal is going to experience personal distress as well as finding him or herself in the middle of considerable staff conflict'.

Variation in responses to illness and death

Staff vary greatly in their responses to different illnesses. Some individuals may be particularly stressed by, or enjoy working with, the articulate demanding teenager; others with the dependent, multihandicapped child; others with the helpless baby requiring technically sophisticated care. Diversity of interest and skills amongst staff is essential for spreading the load, maximizing skills, and minimizing stress.

Concerning different deaths, staff in our hospice study frequently described how distressing a sudden, unexpected, difficult, inconsolable death can be—as indeed can the case of a child who lives beyond the point where he or she was expected to die. Circumstances where the timing or nature of the death defeats preparation and readiness seem to be the crucial factor here. For many, it is particularly distressing to witness the decline of a child who no longer recognizes others and where there is no perceived quality of life. Staff in our study also reported how distressing it could be to be excluded from the care of a dying child for whom they had long been central carers.

Conflict of interest

A dilemma increasingly faced by hospice staff is that of balancing the use of ever more sophisticated life-prolonging equipment with the preservation of quality of life for a child. Staff not infrequently find themselves caring for children discharged home on high dependency equipment such as ventilators, and in the context of very poor quality of life are deeply concerned by the question 'at what cost do we preserve life?'. This is particularly hard when the promotion of patient comfort and dignity lie at the heart of the hospice philosophy of care.

Painful communication

It is easy to underestimate how hard it can be to cope with getting close to children who share their feelings and worries about illness and even about their ultimate death; yet such communication may be essential for the children's attempt to come to terms with what is happening to them. Staff may be greatly helped where their training has included some knowledge about child development and the levels of understanding appropriate to different age groups. This problem is highlighted for night staff, who, in the isolation of the early hours of the morning may be confronted with a deeply distressed child, fearful of his or her illness and possible death. An ill friend may be dying, or may even have died leaving the nearby bed empty. These night staff often miss out on the daytime individual or group support, and may yet carry the weight of a child's distress made all the heavier because it is unshared. The solitary but intense fears of the night sometimes pass unrecognized in the business of the day.

Work overload

There are many occupational hazards, particularly work overload. The question immediately arises whether that load is entirely imposed from outside or whether an additional need to be needed or appear as the most competent member of the team is contributing to it. This may be of particular concern where personal relationships with a patient and family extend outside the work situation. A member of staff's own judgement over trying to help may be impaired and the family's expectations may increase unreasonably. The roles and relationships become less clear and resentments may develop.

Sources of stress within the working team

One member of staff may not value another's professional standing, training, or competence; may develop professional or personal rivalry towards another colleague; may feel possessive about a 'special' child or family with whom they are working; may feel undervalued in relation to one or several of the team members; may feel taken for granted. These tend to be issues around self-worth and a staff member's sense of feeling valued by colleagues.

In a hierarchical team structure, particularly where communication is poor and mutual trust is low, decisions taken at a senior level may be resented, misunderstood, or appear blatantly unreasonable. Senior staff may then be resented and become isolated and unsupported (they too need support). Junior staff left to witness and cope with deeply distressing situations such as the anger, outrage, and anguish of parents and siblings at the untimely death of their child may feel de-skilled and utterly overwhelmed by their own sense of impotence. If unsupported, their full anger at their own sense of helplessness in the face of inescapable tragedy may be projected on to other staff who they may feel have abandoned them to this situation.

Staff who carry unresolved personal relationship problems may, without realizing, seek inappropriately to fill that personal gap with one or more of their professional colleagues. When their needs are not met and demands only responded to by puzzled withdrawal, the reaction may be one of unreasonable anger and criticism. In such cases, it is only too easy for relationship problems that have dogged the individual in the past to be resurrected and re-enacted in relation to one or more colleagues. While the source of the difficulty is not understood, the problem is seen as purely belonging to the present, and can lead to considerable tension.

Conflict may arise because team members have a strong difference of opinion over tackling a particular problem. Any healthy team will encounter many such disputes; Mount and Voyer (1980) have pointed out that any group claiming to work as a team should show their battle scars: 'If they don't have them they haven't worked as a team.' Individual attitudes towards disagreements will determine whether a conflict within the team hardens and becomes disruptive, or becomes part of healthy growth and professional development. For instance, a team member—particularly difficult if a senior member—may view disagreements as intrinsically bad, with differences of opinion taken as personal criticisms rather than professional dialogue. A disagreement interpreted personally can become a destructive conflict.

Those who experience disagreement as a personal threat, a disturbing uncomfortable event, may use a defensive tactic by avoiding it at all costs. Disputes are swept under the carpet, and this often leads to a build-up of tension which can eventually erupt in an untimely and explosive way. Such protection at any cost in team members replicates the frequently described protective defence that operates in some families with terminally ill children (Bluebond-Langner 1978) where child and parents continue a mutual pretence that the illness is not fatal, each side protecting the other from pain, but in so doing driving themselves into isolated positions where a sense of distance and abandonment come to prevail.

Another defence may arise where, in order to avoid facing a difficulty, one member of the team is blamed and scapegoated for all ills. A problem is neatly and inappropriately put into another's lap. The question of where difficulties really do belong is crucial. A good supportive mechanism at work within the team will help to keep communication open and the will to resolve these questions alive.

There are some problems which apply particularly to general practitioners, district nurses, health visitors, and others with large and varied case-loads in primary care. Resentment may build up between colleagues if, for example, one 'special' family with a terminally ill child takes up so much of one colleague's time that he or she may be unable to carry the normal share of work. This may be exacerbated by the family making unrealistic demands, such as insisting on seeing only that member of the team to the exclusion of others and frequently phoning him or her at home, when not on duty. On occasion this may be compounded by a family having rejected some of the team as part of their angry response to the diagnosis. Ultimately this can lead to a wide range of damaging feelings; professional jealousy, frustration, rejection, isolation, feeling overburdened and guilty.

SYMPTOMS OF STRESS

Physical symptoms may be seen as the body responding to 'stress overload' (Vachon and Pakes 1984). It is important once any organic cause has been ruled out, for individual staff to try and recognize the signs of stress in themselves—physical exhaustion, abdominal pain, headache—and to try and avoid the occupational hazard of caring for everyone else while neglecting themselves. Eating healthily, regularly, and not always hurriedly and on the move, having enough exercise and regular sleep; these are obvious but often ignored prerequisites for maintaining physical health and emotional homeostasis. Levels of staffing and the organization of on call and rota systems also crucially affect whether an individual can eat and sleep regularly, and take adequate time off to be with family and friends, and to pursue outside interests.

Psychological symptoms including feelings of depression, sadness, and anxiety commonly occur in sensitive people as normal reactions to highly stressful situations. It is important that such feelings should be acknowledged and not disregarded, and if they do not resolve, help should be sought. At some point most staff will find themselves over-identifying with a particular patient in a way which hinders their ability to help, or feeling suddenly very vulnerable after several deaths have occurred on a unit, or feeling so drained that self-esteem and belief in their own professional competence are threatened. Discussion with colleagues or, where appropriate, in a support group may help restore the perspective. If difficulties go unacknowledged, staff are in danger of unproductive reactions such as flight into constant activity or blotting the problem out with alcohol or other drugs. An inability to detach oneself from the job spells danger and requires scheduling time away from work. It is also unwise for staff constantly to bring job tensions home in the expectation of unlimited support. They risk draining their own family members, who may come to feel that their own needs and interests are ignored and that the quality of ordinary family life is diminished.

MITIGATION AND MANAGEMENT OF STRESS

In a recent review of research on staff stress in hospice/palliative care Mary Vachon points out that stress appears to be less where mechanisms such as social support, involvement in work and decision-making, and a realistic work-load are in place. She argues that the early recognition of the potential areas of stress and the development of appropriate coping strategies probably accounts for the lower than expected stress levels reported across many hospice/palliative care settings (Vachon 1995b).

Staff selection

An applicant's motivation and expectations of working with terminally ill children and their families should be explored. Any recent or previous experience of the death of a relative or close friend, and whether it is likely to be a help or, if unresolved, a hindrance to the job is important. It is relevant to know whether the applicant has a reasonable support system outside work in the form of family, friends, and interests, and whether he or she perceives the significance of these. Candidates should show some self-awareness of their own coping capacities and acknowledge that there will be distress to shoulder. Difficulties are more likely to arise in the case of isolated individuals with a deep need to be needed, who may try to adopt the working team, or the patient and family as substitute friends or family.

The structure of the group

In order to keep stress within manageable levels, much thought and planning needs to be put into the way the working group is structured and run. This is likely to enable stress to be dealt with when it arises and staff to feel supported. In this connection Lansdown *et al.* (1990) discuss stress reduction on a cancer ward.

It is much easier to deal with difficulties at an early stage through established and trusted channels than to be forced in a rearguard action to face a crisis where tension has built up to such a pitch that many staff are leaving, frequently on sick leave, or disaffected and preoccupied with rumbling discontent. Some provision should be built in to the system to care for the carers, and this must be acknowledged as important by senior staff; if they deny the need or block that care then it will fail.

Possible individual and group support systems are discussed in the next section in more detail, but we would emphasize that systems are more effective if problem-airing and problem-solving constitute only a part of their function. If they are used to keep communication in the working group open, they can be a live means of developing professional practice and helping the service evolve so as to meet changing needs. If they are also used as a means of recognizing and affirming good practice, this ensures that such practice does not go unacknowledged but gets built in to the care system.

No matter how the working unit or caring system is set up—whether hierarchical, democratic, formal, or informal—

the importance of the security and flexibility of senior staff cannot be overestimated. Relationships amongst staff with senior members in the team can provide vital support but can also be a source of considerable stress. Senior staff who are not in touch with the experiences of colleagues working on a daily basis with the children and their families may find it difficult to support them adequately and to help them set reasonable limits. The unit head or senior staff members set the tone, working standards, and expectations; and above all, by their behaviour, model a valuing supportive atmosphere. A secure and balanced personality is much better able to set up the trust that will, in turn, draw the support that senior members themselves need in order to survive and thrive. The selection of suitable senior staff is therefore crucial.

The staff member who works alone much of the time and whose 'team' may consist of those colleagues each from a different workplace with whom home support for a family is being managed, is in a more difficult position for getting support for him or herself. The direct line manager may be a busy nursing officer who is rarely seen, administers but cannot support. Seeking out a sympathetic colleague, perhaps arranging regular working lunches to share common practice and concerns is likely to help, for it is much easier to share a major worry or problem with a familiar trusted colleague who already knows one's strengths. Perhaps well-established units, paediatric teams, and hospices should think of inviting more isolated colleagues in, on a regular basis to share support as well as learning from each other's practice.

Training

Training plays a crucial role in helping staff in their professional development, in updating their knowledge and practice, and in improving their communication skills and understanding of interpersonal dynamics—all of which are so vital for understanding the families they serve. Time out and funding for conferences or more extended courses, helps to refresh staff and restore their energies and interest, and in the long run may be highly cost effective. Continued training should not be seen as an additional luxury but as an essential ingredient in maintaining good creative practice and minimizing the sense of impotence and helplessness.

Formal and informal support within the team

There are three advantages in allowing staff as a group the time and means to understand and tackle the difficult issues that necessarily arise in any flourishing team. Firstly, their increased understanding of interpersonal dynamics and pitfalls will be of great benefit in furthering their understanding of the very families they serve. Secondly, while some may argue that teams are really too busy helping families to waste time on the unnecessary nicety of promoting understanding, we would argue to the contrary that time is saved. Prolonged and unresolved staff conflict saps and debilitates the individual and undermines his or her self-esteem, commitment, and efficiency. At its worst, it leads to a rapid changeover of staff with consequent discontinuity of service for child and family. Thirdly, problems and difficulties encountered by those facing great distress have a way of echoing and reverberating in the service set up to help them, with the danger that a service inadvertently mirrors, and therefore reinforces, the very difficulties it aims to ease.

Informal support

Informal support between colleagues in the working team is frequently cited by staff as a major support factor both personally and professionally (Woolley *et al.* 1989). At the same time, conflicts occurring within the team are often cited as a major cause of great distress. Those very individual and group relationships within the working team that can be the greatest sources of support also have the potential to become the focus of the greatest stress and disruption. If staff are aware of possible sources of conflict, they are better able to understand what is happening, identify the real cause of their distress, and avoid conflict reactions. The twin aims with informal support must be to maximize support and minimize stress.

Alongside such informal colleague support, there are other support structures which may be useful for particular teams (Richman 1989).

Regular staff group meeting

Many teams share some form of regular business meeting, ward round, or team meeting, that allows time to review happenings, to discuss developments, air differences, and agree present and future programmes. It is the forum which should lend an ear to any and every member of staff, and all should be encouraged to find a voice at some point in the proceedings. Most people, however, will have experienced regular staff meetings where everything seems to have been discussed but nothing of import actually said; meetings where the tricky issues are neatly avoided, some indeed being too threatening or dangerous to open up between a group of people who must continue their daily work together. This is where other more formal support and help can be useful.

Formal support group

One form of support can be through a regular formal group led by a suitably trained professional who establishes a link with the team but is not a full member on a daily basis. Feelings can run high about whether such a group should exist. Should all team members be expected to attend? Does such an expectation create a threat or intrusion? What professional standing should the leader have? Should the leader be entirely separate from the working team or in some way a part of it? As work settings vary so widely in structure and style, and the personalities differ we would argue for flexibility of approach, each unit having the opportunity to evolve a group to suit its own needs, that is workable, comfortable, and the least threat to the team members. The group is then an organism evolved from within rather than imposed from without. Some individuals intensely dislike the idea of a formal group and may initially find it threatening and difficult to attend; but if colleagues recognize this discomfort and do not press for active participation while valuing that colleague's attendance, even the most unwilling participant may draw support and, in time, join in.

Fears may arise from the belief that the leader will 'analyse' the members in public, open up threatening topics, or somehow undermine confidence by making suggestions inappropriate to the working team's needs. Added to this may be a belief that no professional should need to call in an 'outsider' to sort out problems. These concerns may be avoided if the purpose of the group is carefully thought out when it is set up by participants—though it will redefine itself as it develops—and it is seen as a support group, helped by a sympathetic independent leader to draw out and identify the strengths of their own working practice. The leader is essentially an enabler and carries no executive authority, but in order to be helpful needs knowledge of the team's structure, its aims, and its style of work. As Alexander (1993) points out, without careful consideration of the group's aims, ground rules and leadership, 'the mere aggregation of staff may be neither a group nor a source of support.'

It is perhaps helpful to be sure about what such a support group is not. It is not a teaching seminar. It is not a group analytic dissection exercise. It is not a forum for bypassing the proper authorities and making executive decisions that belong elsewhere. It is not an exercise in scapegoating absent members.

Staff attending a well-established group that meets weekly have stated how useful and important it is to have a regular time set aside, apart from the hectic daily routine, to sit together and review what has happened, to recognize where working practice went well, and to share the weight of particularly difficult or distressing situations. It has also been noted that such meetings can be painful and uncomfortable at times, that enjoyment is quite different from usefulness, and that the sessions which tackle the more difficult and uncomfortable issues sometimes turn out to be the most useful. Senior staff regularly participating in a group can use it also as a primary source of support, because it provides them with the opportunity to air weightier problems in an engaged forum, and when difficult decisions do have to be made, staff may at least understand even if they do not totally agree.

Over time, the group leader is able to highlight the changes and developments which staff from the inside of their daily routine may not necessarily recognize or fully appreciate. The airing of points of difference comes to be safer over time, and where necessary these can be transformed, through the mediation of the leader, from potential personal disputes to professional debate.

Individual support

There will always be some personal issues which are not appropriate to bring to a group meeting, for example when a personal problem is interfering with work. Team members may talk informally with a colleague and most daily difficulties are likely to be dealt with in this way. Where this is not sufficient, it is useful to have an independent consultant/ therapist/counsellor, available on a regular or occasional basis, in order to see staff members in private. The support worker needs to be trusted by the team, and sympathetic to their situation and working aims. He or she should not be seen as the solver of all problems, but a partner with time and experience to enable staff to find their own ways of resolving difficulties.

Issues frequently brought forward concern situations where staff have found themselves unexpectedly responding immoderately to a situation perhaps born of an echo from a past experience which continues to distress them. Discussing these issues and recognizing the cause can give enormous relief and release the staff member to a more even perspective. Feelings of worthlessness may arise at being unable to meet all perceived needs, even those way outside the remit of the working setting. Issues (such as those discussed on p. 171) concerning relationships within the working group may need some careful discussion and gentle unravelling.

Some staff may feel continually 'spent', but have invested all their energies in the job and so feel a sense of guilt about the prospect of leaving or moving on. Encouragement to set limits, pursue outside interests and friendships, even to think of moving on as a positive professional step rather than an admission of personal failure may well be necessary. Paradoxically in a service which constantly tries to help families confront the issue of leave-taking and moving on, it is not unusual for staff to deny themselves the very opportunity to do either.

CONCLUSION

Each working unit will have its own needs, styles of coping, and staff personalities; and setting up supports on an individual or group basis can feel somewhat threatening and awkward. One way to develop a relevant support system is to start by asking all staff about stresses, job satisfaction, and coping strategies, so that everyone has a say in identifying needs and evolving appropriate solutions. Further studies to measure the impact of staff support programmes on improving patient/family care would be invaluable here (Vachon 1995a). Our experience to date suggests that where reasonable supports exist job satisfaction increases, professional practice and development is aided, and the danger of prolonged sick-leave and high staff turnover is lessened. Most important of all, staff contentment and fulfilment reflects in a richer service to families.

ACKNOWLEDGEMENTS

We would like to thank those staff working with terminally ill children and their families whose frank and open discussions have so helped us in the formulation of our ideas. We are extremely grateful to Dr Gillian Forrest and Prof. David Baum for their research collaboration, to Sally Hope and Ede Anthem for their valuable comments and to Sandra Cooper for assistance in preparing the manuscript.

REFERENCES

Alexander, D. A. (1993). Staff support groups: do they support and are they even groups? *Palliative Medicine*, **7**, 127–32.
Bluebond-Langner, M. (1978). *The private worlds of dying children*. Princeton University Press, New Jersey.

Dent, H. S., Gillard, J. H., Aarons, E. J., Crimlisk, H. L., and Smyth-Pigott, P. J. (1990). Preregistration house officers in the four Thames regions: I. Survey of education and workload. *British Medical Journal*, **300**, 713–15.

Jacques, E. (1955). Social systems as a defence against persecutory and depressive anxiety. In *New directions in psychoanalysis*, (ed. M. Klein, P. Heimanne, and R. E. Money-Kyrle). Tavistock, London.

Kubler-Ross, E. (1970). *On death and dying*. Macmillan, New York.

Lansdown, R., Pike, S., and Smith, M. (1990). Reducing stress in the cancer ward. *Nursing Times*, **38**, 34–8.

Lattanzi, M. E. (1985). An approach to caring: caregiver concerns. In *Hospice approaches to pediatric care*, (ed. C. A. Corr and M. C. Corr), pp. 261–77. Springer, New York.

Maguire, P. (1985). Barriers to psychological care of the dying. *British Medical Journal*, **291**, 1171–3.

Menzies-Lyth, I. (1960). A case study in the functioning of social systems as a defence against anxiety. *Human Relations*, **13**, 1–26.

Mount, B. M. and Voyer, S. (1980). Staff stress in palliative hospice care. In *The Royal Victoria Hospital manual on palliative hospice care*, (ed. I. Ajemian and B. M. Mount), p. 446. Arno Press, New York.

Richman, J. M. (1989). Groupwork in a hospice setting. *Social Work with Groups*, **12**, 171–84.

Stein, A. and Woolley, H. (1990). An evaluation of hospice care for children. In *Listen. My child has a lot of living to do*, (ed. J. D. Baum, F. Dominica, and R. Woodward), pp. 66–90. Oxford University Press.

Vachon, M. L. S. (1979). Staff stress in care of the terminally ill. *Quality Review Bulletin*, **5**, 13–17.

Vachon, M. L. S. and Pakes, E. (1984). Staff stress in the care of the critically ill and dying child. In *Childhood and death*, (ed. H. Wass and C. A. Corr), pp. 151–82. Hemisphere Publication Corporation, Washington.

Vachon, M. L. S. (1987). *Occupational stress in the care of the critically ill, the dying, and the bereaved*. Hemisphere Publication Corporation, Washington.

Vachon, M. L., Kristjanson, L., and Higginson, I. (1995a). Psychosocial issues in palliative care: the patient, the family, and the process and outcome of care. *Journal of Pain and Symptom Management*, **10**, 142–50.

Vachon, M. L. (1995b). Staff stress in hospice/palliative care: a review. *Palliative Medicine*, **9**, 92–122.

Woolley, H., Stein, A., Forrest, G. C., and Baum, J. D. (1989). Staff stress and job satisfaction at a children's hospice. *Archives of Disease in Childhood*, **64**, 114–18.

Appendix A
Drug list

Drug	Total daily dose	Times daily	Notes
Amitryptyline			
Oral	0.5 mg/kg	At night	This is low dose, for nerve pain.
	1–2 mg/kg	3	Antidepressant dose.
Preparations:			
mixture	10 mg in 5 ml		
tablets	10 mg, 25 mg, or 50 mg		
Baclofen			
Oral	0.5–2 mg/kg	2–3	Increase dose gradually; maximum 80 mg daily; decrease dose in renal failure.
Preparations:			
liquid	5 mg in 5 ml		
tablets	10 mg		
Benztropine			
Oral	0.1 mg/kg	2–3	For drug-induced extra pyramidal symptoms.
Intravenous	0.1 mg/kg (max. 2 mg)		
Preparations:			
tablets	2 mg		
injection	1 mg/1 ml		

Drug	Total daily dose	Times daily	Notes
Bisacodyl			
Oral, Rectal	5 mg	1	Stimulant laxative. Doses and frequency can be increased; acts in 12 hr oral, 20–60 min rectal.
Preparations:			
tablets	5 mg		
suppositories	5 mg, 10 mg		
Carbamazepine			
Oral	10–20 mg/kg	2–3	For nerve pain; increase to maintenance dose gradually.
Preparations:			
liquid	100 mg/5 ml		
tablets	100 mg, 200 mg, or 400 mg		
Chlorpheniramine			
Oral	200–400 μg/kg	3–4	
Intravenous	200 μg/kg	Single dose	
Preparations:			
syrup	2 mg/5 ml		
tablets	4 mg		
injection	10 mg/ml		
Codeine phosphate			
Oral	1–3 mg/kg	4–6	Antidiarrhoea, antitussive.
	3–6 mg/kg	4–6	Analgesic.
Preparations:			
linctus	15 mg/5 ml		
	3 mg/5 ml		
syrup	25 mg/5 ml		
tablets	15 mg, 30 mg		
Cyclizine			
Oral, Rectal	< 1 year, 1 mg/kg/dose	3	Particularly for emesis of raised intracranial pressure.
	1–4 years, 12.5 mg/dose	3	
	4–12 years, 25 mg/dose	3	
	> 12 years, 50 mg/dose	3	

Drug	Total daily dose	Times daily	Notes
Cyclizine *(cont.)*			
Subcutaneous	Total daily dose as above		Compatible with diamorphine for infusion.
Preparations:			
tablets	50 mg		
suppositories	25 mg by special request		
injection	50 mg/ml (can be given orally)		
Danthron (Co-danthramer)			
Oral	2.5–5 ml (of 25/200)	1–2	Stimulant. Acts in 6–12 hr; increase dose if needed; may make urine red.
Preparations:			
suspension	25/200 in 5 ml		
strong susp.	75/1000 in 5 ml		
Dantrolene			
Oral	1 mg/kg	1	Starting dose, increase gradually to 12 mg/kg/day in three doses.
Preparations:			
capsules	25 mg, 100 mg		
Dexamethasone			
Oral	2–10 mg	2	Reduces tumour swelling; use minimum dose for effect; short course and taper dose.
Preparations:			
tablets	0.5 mg, 2 mg		
injections	4 mg/ml, can be given orally		
Diamorphine			
Intravenous/ subcutaneous	20 μg/kg/hr continuous or 1/3 total 24 hr oral dose of morphine sulphate over 24 hr		Used in infusions because of greater solubility than morphine.
Preparations:			
ampoules	5 mg, 10 mg, 30 mg, 100 mg, 500 mg		Tablets available but no advantage over morphine.

Drug	Total daily dose	Times daily	Notes
Diazepam			
Oral	500 μg	3	Anxiolytic and antispasmodic.
Rectal	1–3 years, 5 mg 4–12 years, 10 mg	Single dose	Anticonvulsant. Repeat if needed.
Intravenous	250 μg/kg	Single dose	Anticonvulsant. Slow intravenous over 3 min; repeat if needed in 5 min.
	100 μg/kg/hr	Continuous	Starting dose after bolus.
Preparations:			
tablets	2 mg, 5 mg, 10 mg		
syrup	2 mg/5 ml, 5 mg/5 ml		
rectal tubes	5 mg, 10 mg in 2.5 ml		
suppositories	10 mg		
injection	10 mg/2 ml (500 μg in 0.1 ml)		
Diclofenac			
Oral, Rectal	1–3 mg/kg	3	Slow release once daily.
Preparations:			
tablets	25 mg, 50 mg		
dispersable	50 mg		
slow release	75 mg, 100 mg		
suppositories	12.5 mg, 25 mg, 50 mg, 100 mg		
Dihydrocodeine			
Oral	< 4 years, 500 μg/kg > 4 years, 1–2 mg/kg/dose	4–6	Prescribe laxative.
Preparations:			
tablets	30 mg		
elixir	10 mg/5 ml (contains alcohol)		
Docusate sodium			
Oral	5 mg/kg	1–3	Stimulant/softener.
Rectal	< 3 years 2.5 ml > 3 years 5 ml		Large initial doses and reduce; dilute with milk or orange; oral acts in 1–2 days.
Preparations:			
capsules	100 mg		
elixir	12.5 mg, 50 mg in 5 ml		
enema	5 ml		

Drug	Total daily dose	Times daily	Notes
Domperidone			
Oral	1–2 mg/kg	3–6	
Rectal	2–4 mg/kg	3–6	
Preparations:			
tablets	10 mg		
suspension	1 mg/ml		
suppositories	30 mg		
Fluconazole			
Oral	3 mg/kg	1	For 7–14 days for mucosal candidiasis
Preparations:			
capsules	50 mg, 150 mg		
suspension	50 mg/5 ml, 200 mg/5 ml		
Haloperidol			
Oral	1–12 years 25–50 µg/kg	2	
	> 12 years, 3 mg	2	
Subcutaneous	25–50 µg/kg	Continuous	Compatible with diamorphine.
Preparations:			
tablets	1.5 mg, 5 mg, 10 mg, 20 mg		
capsules	500 ug		
liquid	2 mg/ml		
injection	5 mg/ml, 20 mg/2 ml		
Hyoscine butylbromide (antispasmodic)			
Subcutaneous	600–1200 µg/kg/24 hr		Compatible with diamorphine.
Preparations:			
injection	20 mg/ml		
Hyoscine hydrobromide (to decrease bronchial secretion)			
Transdermal	< 4 years, ½ patch		
	> 4 years, 1 patch		
Subcutaneous	30–60 µg/kg/ 24 hr	Continuous	Compatible with diamorphine.

Drug	Total daily dose	Times daily	Notes
Hyoscine hydrobromide *(cont.)*			
Preparations:			
transdermal (Scopaderm patch)	500 µg/72 hr		
injection	400 µg/ml, 600 µg/ml		
Ibuprofen			
Oral	20 mg/kg	3	Modified release preparations available.
Preparations:			
tablets	200 mg, 400 mg, 600 mg		
suspension	100 mg/5 ml		
Lactulose			
Oral	1 ml/kg	1–2	Osmotic laxative. Starting dose, adjust according to response; acts over 24 hr.
Preparations:			
solution	3.5 g/5 ml		
Loperamide			
Oral	200 µg/kg	3–4	Higher doses have been used.
Preparations:			
capsules	2 mg		
syrup	1 mg/5 ml		
Methotrimeprazine			
Oral	250 µg–1 mg/kg/dose	3–6	Sedative and antiemetic. In adults much lower doses (5 mg/24 hrs) have been used for antiemesis alone.
Subcutaenous	500 µg–3 mg/kg/24 hr	Continuous	Compatible with diamorphine for infusion.
Preparations:			
tablets	25 mg		
injection	25 mg/ml		

Drug	Total daily dose	Times daily	Notes
Metoclopramide			
Oral Intravenous Subcutaneous	300–500 μg/kg	3 Continuous	For emesis with chemotherapy up to 0.5 mg/kg/dose as intravenous bolus; dystonic reactions can occur at any dose, reversed with benztropine, compatible with diamorphine for infusion.

Preparations:
  tablets
  solution
  injection
	10 mg
	1 mg/ml
	5 mg/ml		

Micro-enema (sodium citrate)			
Rectal	5 ml disposable pack		Acts in 15–30 mins.
Midazolam			
Subcutaneous	250 μg–1 mg/kg/24 hr	Continuous	Lower dose for anxiolysis, higher dose and increase if needed for anticonvulsant and sedation.
Preparations: injection	2 mg/ml, 5 mg/ml		
Morphine sulphate			
Oral, Rectal	< 1 year, 1 mg/kg > 1 year, 2 mg/kg > 12 years, 60 mg	6 for short acting 2 for slow release (MST)	Starting doses and increase for analgesia. Decrease dose in renal failure. With slow release always provide short acting opioid for breakthrough pain. Can use slow release tablets rectally.

Drug	Total daily dose	Times daily	Notes
Morphine sulphate *(cont.)*			
Preparations:			
Oromorph mixture	10 mg/5 ml, 100 mg/5 ml		
tablets	10 mg, 20 mg, 50 mg		
suppositories	10 mg, 15 mg, 20 mg, 30 mg		
MST tablets	5 mg, 10 mg, 15 mg, 30 mg, 60 mg, 100 mg, 200 mg		
MST suspension	20 mg, 30 mg, 60 mg, 100 mg, 200 mg		
Naproxen			
Oral, Rectal	10 mg/kg	2–3	
Preparations:			
tablets	250 mg, 375 mg, 500 mg		
suspension	125 mg/5 ml		
suppositories	500 mg		
Ondansetron			
Oral	< 4 years, 2 mg/dose	2–3	
	> 4 years, 4 mg/dose	2–3	
	Adult, 8 mg	2–3	
Preparations:			
tablets	4 mg, 8 mg		
Paraldehyde			
Rectal	0.3 ml/kg max. 10 ml		Mix with equal volume of arachis or olive oil; insert immediately if plastic syringe used; repeat 1–2 hourly if needed.
Preparations:			
injection	5 ml, 10 ml		
Phenobarbitone			
Intravenous	15 mg/kg	Single dose	Slow injection over 5 min.
Subcutaneous	500 μg/kg/hr	Continuous	Increase as needed, use separate infusion.
Preparations:			
injection	30 mg/ml, 60 mg/ml, 200 mg/ml		

Drug	Total daily dose	Times daily	Notes
Prochloreperazine			
Oral, Rectal	250 µg/kg/dose	2–3	Not suitable for subcutaneous infusion as it is a skin irritant.
Preparations:			
syrup	1 mg/ml		
tablets	5 mg, 25 mg		
suppositories	5 mg, 25 mg		
Propantheline			
Oral	1–2 mg	2–3	
Preparations:			
tablets	15 mg		
segments	3.75 mg, 7.5 mg		
Senna			
Oral	< 2 years, 1.25–2.5 ml	1	Stimulant. Acts in 8–12 hrs.
	2–6 years, 2.5–5 ml		
	½–1 tablet		
	> 6 years, 5–10 ml		
	1–2 tablets		
Preparations:			
tablets	7.5 mg		
syrup	7.5 mg/5 ml		
Tranexamic acid			
Oral	90 mg/kg	3	
Mouthwash		3	Can use intravenous solution orally.
Preparations:			
tablets	500 mg		
syrup	500 mg/5 ml		

Appendix B
Useful contacts

This is only a selection of organizations; more comprehensive lists of information are available from ACT, Contact-A-Family, and the National AIDS Helpline.

ACT (Association for children with life threatening or terminal conditions and their families)

Umbrella organization for professionals and parents. Links statutory, charitable and self-help groups. Information service, education.
65 St Michael's Hill, Bristol BS2 8DZ. Tel: (01179) 221556.

Alder Centre

Drop-in centre and other services for all those affected by the death of a child.
Alder Hey Children's Hospital NHS Trust, Eaton Road, Liverpool L12 2AP. Tel: (0151) 252 5391.

Barnardos

A number of support services for children with life-threatening illnesses, some of which include bereavement support. Tel: (0181) 550 8822.

Childline

Counselling for any child with any problem; 24 hr. Free and confidential. Tel: (0800) 1111.

Child Death Helpline

For anyone affected by the death of a child. All calls answered by parents who have themselves lost a child. Based at Great Ormond Street Children's Hospital NHS Trust, Great Ormond Street, London WC1N 3JH and Alder Centre, Alder Hey Children's Hospital NHS Trust, Eaton Road, Liverpool L12 2AP. Open 7.00 p.m.–10.00 p.m. every day and Monday, Wednesday and Friday 10.00 a.m.–1.00 p.m. Freephone 0800 282986.

The Children's Trust

Respite care, rehabilitation, care of chronic sick, and terminal care.
Tadworth Court, Tadworth, Surrey KT20 5RU. Tel: (01737) 357171.

Compassionate Friends

A self-help group for parents who have lost a child of any age. Support locally, leaflets, and a postal library available.
53 North Street, Bedminster, Bristol BS3 1EN. Tel: (01179) 539639.

Contact-A-Family

National charity for parents of children born with special needs; providing advice, support, and links with local and national groups for specific or rare conditions. Information for professionals also.
170 Tottenham Court Road, London W1P 0HA. Tel: (0171) 383 3555.

Cruse

National bereavement care organization.
126 Sheen Road, Richmond, Surrey. Tel: (0181) 940 4818.
Helpline Tel: (0181) 332 7227.

CLIC (Cancer and Leukaemia in Childhood Trust)

Charity focused on treatment, welfare, and research for children with malignant disease. Newsletter.
CLIC House, 12–13 King Street, Bristol BS2 8JH. Tel: (0117) 9248844.

Cystic Fibrosis Research Trust

Charity financing research and treatment, support and advice to families with cystic fibrosis. Leaflets available. Newsletter.
11 London Road, Bromley, Kent BR1 1BY. Tel: (0181) 464 7211.

Genetics Interest Group (GIG)

Organization to improve services for people with genetic disorders. Helpline and regional links. Newsletter.
Farringdon Point, 29–35 Farringdon Road, London EC1M 3JB. Tel: (0171) 430 0090.

Heartline Association

For parents of children born with heart disease. Support literature and bereavement group.
Rossmore House, 26 Park Street, Camberley, Surrey GU15 3PL. Tel: (01276) 675655.

Hospices for children

For list of hospices currently, or imminently open contact ACT (address as before).

Leukaemia Care Society

Support through information, financial help and holidays for those with leukaemia and allied blood disorders.
14 Kingfisher Court, Vinny Bridge, Pinhoe, Devon EX4 8JN. Tel: (01392) 464848.

Leukaemia Research Fund

Supports research. Information booklets for parents. Newsletter.
43 Great Ormond Street, London WC1N 3JH. Tel: (0171) 405 0101.

Meditec

Specialized book service for professionals and families. Booklist, mail order service. All aspects of dying, etc.
Meditec, Jackson's Yard, Brewery Hill, Grantham, Lincs NG31 6DW. Tel: (01476) 590505.

The Multiple Births Foundation (MBF)

For professional support of families with twins and higher order births. Includes bereavement support.
Queen Charlotte's & Chelsea Hospital, Goldhawk Road, London W6 0XG. Tel: (0181) 383 3519.

Muscular Dystrophy Group of Great Britain and Northern Ireland

Funds research, care, education for professionals and families, leaflets. Newsletter.
7–11 Prescott Place, London SW4 6BS. Tel: (0171) 720 8055.

Nigel Clare Network Trust (NCNT)

Aims to improve quality of life for families with child with reduced life expectancy; emphasis on helping preserve parental employment and retraining, to reduce financial hardship.
85 Moorgate, London EC2M 6SA. Tel: (0171) 256 8313.

Royal Association for Disability and Rehabilitation (RADAR)

12 City Forum, 250 City Road, London EC1V 8AF. Tel: (0171) 250 3222.

REACT (Research, Education and Aid for Children with Terminal Disease)

Assists families with unexpected financial needs.
St Luke's House, 270 Sandycombe Road, Kew, Richmond, Surrey TW9 3NP. Tel: (0181) 940 2575.

RTMCD (Research Trust for Metabolic Diseases in Children)

Research, parent information, and support; 24 hr helpline for newly diagnosed and bereaved. Newsletter.
Golden Gate Lodge, Weston Road, Crewe, Cheshire CW1 1XM. Tel: (01270) 250221.

SANDS (Stillbirths and Neonatal Deaths)

Bereavement support for families when a baby is stillborn or dies shortly after birth.
28 Portland Place, London W1N 4DE. Helpline: Tel: (0171) 436 5881.

Sargent Cancer Care for Children

Financial help for families, fund social workers for paediatric oncology.
14 Abingdon Road, London W8 6AF. Tel: (0171) 565 5100.

TAMBA (Twins and multiple birth association)

For parents with twins and multiple births including bereavement support.
PO Box 30, Little Sutton, South Wirral L66 1TH. (0151) 348 0020.

Wish-granting organizations

There are several organizations offering to grant wishes for seriously ill children. Addresses can be found in the booklet *Children with cancer–guide to help for families*, from ACT.

HIV/AIDS ORGANIZATIONS

Some organizations are given below. Detailed information available through the National AIDS Helpline.

National AIDS Helpline

Information and advice on all aspects of HIV/AIDS. Free confidential 24 hr line. Freephone 0800 567 123.

Barnardos Positive Options

Supports children and young people who have HIV/AIDS or who are indirectly affected through the illness of their parents.
22 Angel Gate, City Road, London EC1V 2PT. Tel: (0171) 278 5039.

Blackliners

Services include support and counselling to Asian, African, and Afro-Caribbean people affected by HIV/AIDS.
Eurolink Business Centre, 49 Effra Road, London SW2 1BZ. Tel: (0171) 738 5274.

PPC (Positively Partners and Children)

Support for people who are HIV positive, and their partners and family.
Unit F7, Shakespeare Business Centre, 245a Coldharbour Lane, London SW9 8PR. Tel: (0171) 738 7333.

The Terrence Higgins Trust

Information, advice and help on HIV/AIDS.
Helpline Tel: (0171) 242 1010.

Religious Groups

London Churches HIV/AIDS Ecumenical Trust and Forum

Organization in London acting ecumenically in the field of HIV and AIDS, and represents the Baptist Union, Church Army, Church of England, Forum on Afro-Caribbean Churches, Jewish Community, Methodist Church, Catholic Church, Salvation Army, Society of Friends, and the United Reform Church.

St Paul's Church, Lorrimore Square, London SE17 3QU. Tel: (0171) 793 0338.

Appendix C
Books for parents and children

There are many books available both for parents and children, and this is just a small selection. An extensive list and mail order facility is available from Meditec, Jackson's Yard, Brewery Hill, Grantham, Lincs NG31 6DW. Tel. (0476) 590505.

BOOKS FOR PARENTS

ACT (1990). *Children with cancer—guide to help for families.* Booklet available from ACT, Institute of Child Health, Royal Hospital for Sick Children, St Michael's Hill, Bristol BS2 8BJ. Tel: (0272) 221556.

Baum, D., Dominica, F., and Woodward, R. (1990). *Listen. My child has a lot of living to do.* Oxford University Press.

Buckman, R. (1980). *I don't know what to say—how to help and support someone who is dying.* Papermac, London.

Contact-A-Family (1990). *Child disability benefits and other sources of help.* Booklet available from Contact-a-Family, 16 Strutton Ground, London SW1P 2HP. Tel: (071) 222 2695.

Cooper, A. and Halpin, B. (1991). *This is our child—how parents experience the medical world.* Oxford University Press.

Gaffney, D. (1988). *The seasons of grief—helping children grow through loss.* Plume Books, Ontario.

Grollman, E. (1993). *Straight talk about death for teenagers.* Beacon Press, Boston.

Grollman, E. (1996). *Talking about death*. Beacon Press, London.

Schiff, H. S. (1977, reissued 1992). *The bereaved parent*. Souvenir Press, London.

Wilkinson, T. (1991). *The death of a child—a book for families*. Julia MacRae Books, London.

BOOKS FOR CHILDREN

Illness and Treatment

Cancer

Althea. (1989). *I have cancer*. Dinosaur, London.

Bales, H. (1987). *What's up mate*. Hodder & Stoughton, Sevenoaks.

Reuter, E. (1989). *Christopher's story*. Hutchison, London.

Cystic fibrosis

Crollick, A. (1989). *Tell the world*. Video for adolescents available from Cystic Fibrosis Research Trust, Alexandra House, 5 Blyth Road, Bromley, Kent.

Pettenuzzo, B. (1988). *I have cystic fibrosis*. Franklin Watts, London.

Others

Althea. (1982). *I can't talk like you*. Dinosaur, London.

Jessel, C. (1975, reprinted 1978). *Mark's wheelchair adventures*. Methuen Childrens Books, London.

Pettenuzzo, B. (1988). *I have cerebral palsy*. Franklin Watts, London.

Books about death

Althea. *When Uncle Bob died*. Dinosaur, London. Book about the death of a young adult and the child's feelings of grief. No religious philosophy included. Age range 5–8.

Cohn, J. (1987). *I had a friend named Peter*. William Morrow, New York. Beautifully illustrated story in which a little girl learns of the sudden death of her friend. Helpful introduction for parents.

Little, J. (1985). *Mama's going to buy you a mockingbird*. Puffin, Ontario. A sensitive story of a boy's experience and response to his father's illness and death. Age range 10–14.

Mellonie, B. and Inkpen, R. (1983). *Lifetimes*. Paper Tiger, Limpsfield, UK. Illustrated poem with the theme of 'death as part of life' for all living things. Suitable for wide age range and all religious backgrounds.

Miklowitz, G. (1987). *Goodbye tomorrow*. Lion Teen Tracks, Glasgow. A teenager learns he has AIDS. The effects on himself and his family and friends are explored.

Perkins, G. (1996). *Remembering my brother*. A & C Black, London. Story for children with photographs of a real family and their feelings when a brother dies of a brain tumour.

Stickney, D. (1982). *Waterbugs and dragonflies*. A. R. Mowbray, London. Simply written story using the life and development of the dragonfly as an analogy for man's life on earth and life after death. Helpful book for families with a firm belief in an afterlife.

Varley, S. (1984). *Badger's parting gift*. William Collins, London. Illustrated story of the death of an elderly and well-loved badger and how his animal friends come to terms with this. Suitable for all religious backgrounds.

White, E. B. (1952). *Charlotte's web*. Puffin Books, Harmondsworth. Wilbur the pig's life is saved by Charlotte, the wise spider. The end of Charlotte's life is movingly described and the emotions honestly portrayed. For primary school children. Cartoon video version available.

Appendix D
Allowances

Disability Living Allowance

This has two components to help people with the extra costs which arise from care and mobility needs.

The care component of the DLA is paid at three different rates, the higher, the middle, and the lower, depending on the level of help needed by the person claiming. The mobility component (only available for people aged five and over) is available at a higher or lower rate depending on the level of the person's mobility. The condition or conditions entitling a claimant to a care component, a mobility component or both, will have to have existed for three months, although patients considered terminally ill will be able to have their claim met immediately. A special application form is needed for a terminally ill patient (DS1500).

In March 1991, the Department of Health defined the terminally ill as 'Those with an active and progressive disease for which curative treatment is not possible or not appropriate and whose death can reasonably be expected within 12 months'.

The application forms for someone who is not terminally ill, are long and complicated, and a professional helper (e.g. doctor, occupational therapist, or social worker) may need to help the claimant make their application and sign the forms. Professional advice should also be sought by families receiving income support, to assess any extra premium entitlement.

Death Grant

At the time of registration of the death, the registrar can also provide a form (BD8) which will enable a family on Income Support to apply for a grant from the DSS. If families wish to apply for the death grant, they need to take a written estimate from the funeral director and also the documents issued by the registrar, that is, the Certificate for Burial or Cremation, and form BD8 to their local DSS office. Specific charities may also give help towards the cost of a child's funeral. Sargent Cancer Care frequently helps in this manner. If the child has died in hospital and this is some way from the child's home, the hospital may have funds available to help pay for transport back home for the funeral. The hospital social worker may be the best person to know what help is available at this time.

Appendix E
Existing children's hospices in the UK

ACORNS
103 Oak Tree Lane
Selly Oak
Birmingham B29 6HZ
Tel: 0121 628 0210

DERIAN HOUSE
Chancery Road
Astley Village
Chorley, Lancs PR7 1DH
Tel: 01257 233300

EASTERN REGION CHILDREN'S
HOSPICE
Church Lane
Milton
Cambridge CB4 6AB
Tel: 01223 860306

FRANCIS HOUSE
390 Parrs Wood Road
Didsbury
Manchester M20 0NA
Tel: 0161 434 4118

HELEN HOUSE
37 Leopold Street
Oxford, Oxon OX4 1QT
Tel: 01865 728251

HOPE HOUSE
Nant Lane
Morda
Nr. Oswestry
Shrops SY10 9BX
Tel: 01691 671999

LITTLE BRIDGE HOUSE
Redlands Road
Fremington
Barnstaple EX31 2PZ
Tel: 01271 25270

MARTIN HOUSE
Grove Road
Clifford
Wetherby
W. Yorks LS23 6TX
Tel: 01937 845045

NAOMI HOUSE
Stockbridge Road
Sutton Scotney
Winchester
Hants SO21
Tel: 01962 774624

QUIDENHAM CHILDREN'S
HOSPICE
Quidenham
Norwich
Norfolk NR16 2PH
Tel: 01953 888603

RACHEL HOUSE
Avenue Road
Kinross
Scotland KY13 7EP
Tel: 01577 86577

RAINBOWS CHILDREN'S
HOSPICE
Lark Rise, Off Hazel Road
Loughborough
Leicester LE11 2HS
Tel: 0150 923 0800

ZOE'S PLACE
(Baby Hospice)
Life Health Centre
Yew Tree Lane
West Derby
Liverpool L12 9HH
Tel: 0151 228 0353

Index